Mental Health Care

A workbook for carers

Emma Lee

Foreword by Pr

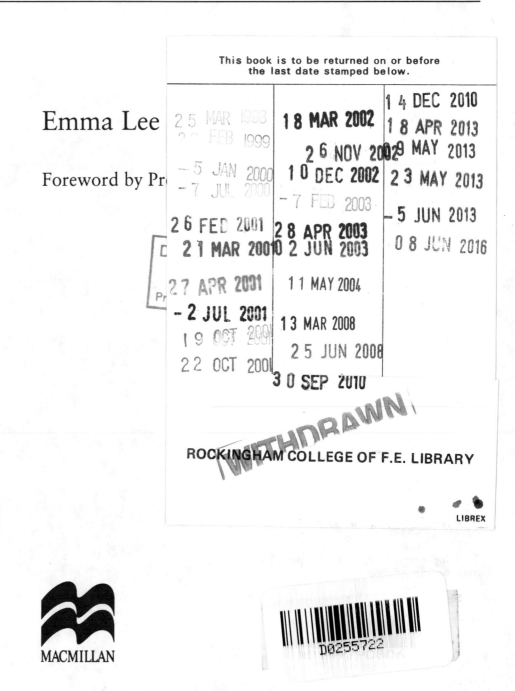

MACMILLAN

For my mother, Emily Videnovic

First published 1997 by
MACMILLAN PRESS LTD
Houndmills, Basingstoke, Hampshire RG21 6XS
and London
Companies and representatives
throughout the world

ISBN 0-333-63757-7

A catalogue record for this book is available
from the British Library

Typeset by ⚡Tek Art, Croydon, Surrey

Printed in Hong Kong

10   9   8   7   6   5   4   3   2   1
06 05 04 03 02 01 00 99 98 97

004998
18/8/97

Contents

Foreword

The past 30 years have seen a transformation in the way in which society responds to the needs and the predicaments of people in psychological turmoil and distress. Where once the main location of treatment was the large, remote and isolated mental hospital, it is now fragmented and scattered among acute psychiatric units in general hospitals, general practitioners' surgeries, social work departments, accident and emergency units, half-way houses and hostels. For some, indeed, there is no location of treatment at all – the number of the mentally ill among the homeless, particularly in the inner cities, is an issue which serves to remind us that we have yet to establish a truly comprehensive system of community care. Where previously the great bulk of those experiencing moderate to severe mental ill-health were hidden behind the grim, forbidding walls of the asylums, separated physically and geographically from the rest of society, now they are part and parcel of modern society with all that that entails.

This transformation brings with it major responsibilities for those working in services delivering mental health care. They are not new responsibilities but they have acquired a sharper and more clearly defined focus. There is a massive need for relevant knowledge and appropriate expertise, for a comprehensive understanding and a range of therapeutic skills. There is a need too for advocacy to help people receive proper treatment, appropriate benefits and adequate support. There is a pressing need for public education to help demystify mental illness and to confront and eliminate stigma and stereotyping. There is a need for political action at local and national level to ensure that the rights of the mentally ill and their carers and the integrity of the mental health services are protected and enhanced.

This extensive workbook provides much-needed information to help care workers address these needs. It summarises in a comprehensive yet concise and lucid fashion the various approaches to mental ill-health, its detection and management, and indicates how the reader can amplify and expand his or her knowledge by appropriate additional reading. The book considers various models, psychiatric and anti-psychiatric, behavioural and psycho-dynamic, personal and group, in a straightforward way without recourse to the awarding of primacy or a hierarchy in terms of effectiveness or usefulness. What the workbook does do is lay out a framework for study and action which should ensure that any care worker who takes the time to read it through will possess at the conclusion of the task a properly informed and balanced understanding of the issues and the challenges involved, of where the boundaries of responsibility are appropriately drawn and where to go when advice is needed and additional expertise required.

Professor Anthony Clare

Acknowledgements

I should like to thank those who have helped at various stages in the preparation of the text, in particular Stuart Sillars, language consultant to the Macmillan Caring Series; Maureen Broomhead, Darlington College; Ralph Verlander and colleagues at Life Opportunities Trust; Sheila Hawkins and Iris Nutting at the Mental After Care Association; and Terry Smyth, Colchester Institute.

All the photographs in the book were taken by Jerry Campbell, whose help I acknowledge with grateful thanks. I should like to thank the Reverend Harry Kudiabor at the Unity Centre in South London for permission to take photographs in the Centre. My thanks also go to Karl Spencer of Sper Consultancy who helped with other photographs.

Thanks are due to the following for permission to use copyright material: King's Fund for the cover of their publication *Power to the People*, Liz Winn (editor), London, 1990 (page 93); Mind (The National Association for Mental Health, 15–19 Broadway, London E15 4BQ) for an extract from their Yellow Card (page 12) and the front cover of the Cantonese version of their leaflet *Understanding Mental Illness* (page 74); the National Schizophrenia Fellowship (28 Castle Street, Kingston-upon-Thames, Surrey KT1 1SS) for the cover of the Gujarati version of their *Notes for Relatives and Friends on Schizophrenia* (page 74). The material reproduced on pages 22 and 28 is Crown copyright.

Every effort has been made to trace all copyright holders, but if any have been inadvertently overlooked the publisher will be pleased to make the necessary arrangements at the first opportunity.

About this book

The effects of community care have brought challenges to care workers, clients and clients' relatives, and to the community as a whole. People with mental health problems are spending less time in hospital and more in the community. An increasing number of individuals with little or no specialist training in mental health find themselves thrown in at the deep end as they face the task of caring for someone with mental health needs, who might have other health care needs as well.

One of the positive things about this is that more people at various levels of care and in a wide range of contexts (from residential mental health settings to family homes) are needed and are being encouraged to care. Often their contribution lies in assisting other mental health workers and care professionals.

This book attempts to help the carer gain the knowledge, understanding and skills needed to be a mental health carer.

Who is the book for?

The book will be of value to you if you are working or training to work in mental health. You could be working full- or part-time, in paid health care, the social services or the voluntary sector, or caring for a member of your family or a friend.

This book will be of special help if you are:

- in training and preparing for assessment for a National Vocational Qualification (NVQ) or Scottish Vocational Qualification (SVQ) in care at level 3, specialising in mental health care. It will also help you if you are studying for an Advanced GNVQ in Health and Social Care.
- employed in a mental health setting and have a job which is supportive to those of other mental health and social care professionals: for example, if you are working as a support worker, social work assistant, welfare assistant or housing officer to social workers, nursing staff (for example, mental health community nurses), officers for mental health settings or occupational therapists within the mental health services. You could also be helping a range of mental health project/community workers on advocacy projects or projects which aim to provide mental health services for particular groups of people, such as those of a different culture, race or gender orientation.
- undertaking social work training (DipSW, CQSW or CSS), especially in the first year. It will also help if you have a social care qualification and wish to update or refresh your knowledge of mental health care, perhaps after a break from work.

- caring for a relative or friend or doing voluntary work where knowledge of mental health care would improve the quality of life of those you care for.

The aims of this book

The book aims to show that mental health care is mostly about learning skills and gaining and applying appropriate knowledge, as well as about building up an understanding of your clients and of yourself.

The underlying aim of the book is to show that mental health care is about developing attitudes and practices that will improve the lives of those who have mental health problems and will truly make them feel valued members of the community.

The scope of the book

The book is mainly about the knowledge and skills necessary for working with adults for whom mental health is the main focus of care. This is not to suggest that caring for someone's mental health is always, if ever, something which could or should be isolated from other needs. For example, your clients' physical well-being, the existing social support, the state of their housing, their work or lack of it, are all interrelated and can influence their mental health.

Difficulties in mental health can and sometimes do appear as one problem among other health problems, such as chronic physical illness. You might be working or training to work with people who have some physical disability, or perhaps learning difficulties, and some clients within these groups might need mental health care as well as other specialist care.

This book cannot cover all these areas of care in detail. The context of the book is a care setting, including clients' homes, for adults who are mostly physically mobile, without major sensory impairment and of average learning ability. The book will be useful to you if you care for people who need other types of care besides that for mental health if you use it together with specialist texts, such as those on caring for older people or young children.

Using the book

This is not a book to be read from cover to cover. You will make best use of it if you go through it carefully, doing the suggested activities where possible and discussing what you do not fully understand with your supervisor and senior colleagues.

- The book is divided into five chapters which can be studied in any sequence to suit your needs. You will see that some sections, such as those on communication, are related, so it makes sense to study these together or in sequence.
- Appendix 1 at the back of the book shows the links between NVQ/SVQ units and different parts of the text. Core units are integrated throughout the book, just as the knowledge and skills to which they relate are used in your work with clients.
- You will learn best and enjoy the process more if you take one step at a time – one section, one activity – and consider all the possible implications to the work you do in your care setting.

About the use of gender

The use of 'he' and 'she' alternates throughout the book and refers to both genders: that is, 'he' is used to mean both he and she, just as 'she' refers to he and she as well. This is to avoid long and awkward sentences which the use of both 'he or she' and 'him/herself' tend to create.

The use of gender in whatever context in this book is not meant to suggest that a particular role (such as that of a client, for example) belongs more to one gender than the other. Any of us, irrespective of gender, has potential for any of the roles referred to in this book, whether it be that of a care worker, a client or something else.

About the names used in this book

All the names used in this book, such as those presented in the activities and examples, and all the events described in those examples, are fictional. They do not bear any relation whatsoever to anyone who may have the same name or names, and they do not relate to any person known to the author but are purely a product of her imagination.

1 Thinking about mental health care

1.1 Images of mental disorder

We all know what it means to be physically healthy. If asked to present a picture of physical health, we might use descriptions such as:

- feeling well, being free from any aches, pains, or discomfort;
- looking healthy (as opposed to looking paler than usual);
- having a healthy appetite and healthy bodily functions;
- having sufficient energy for the daily demands of work and play;
- sleeping well.

Cultural factors

Your image of a mentally distressed individual is likely to be influenced by the views and values of the culture in which you live – that is, what that culture regards as 'normal' feelings and behaviour. The majority of people manage (or appear to manage) to live up to such cultural expectations: for example, to appear sombre and sad, as opposed to happy, during a funeral.

If you attempted the previous activity, you should have come up with a list of feelings and behaviours which you are likely to use as a guide to whether or not someone, or yourself, is feeling mentally distressed.

Image of 'illness'

The phrase *mental illness* is used frequently in our culture, despite the fact that for the great majority of mental health problems there is no scientific evidence that we are talking about illness of a biochemical nature. As you will see in section 1.3, the opinion that mental distress is of biophysical origin is only one of several currently held views.

Due to the popularity of the medical view, one of the images of mental distress is that it is an illness. This image influences the way people are viewed and treated – often as passive receivers of medical care, who need only to do as they are told (in most cases this means taking medication) without much regard for their unique potential to work at overcoming their mental health problems.

However, there are also some positive effects of the image of illness given to mental distress, and these are discussed in section 1.2.

Language used in this book

If you completed the second part of the previous activity, you probably noticed that feelings and behaviour feature predominantly in your description. Because of this, I think it is more appropriate to talk about *mental distress*; this description refers to feelings, such as those of deep sadness, dread, anxiety or an extreme fear. The term *mental disorder* will sometimes also be used because 'disorder' suggests behaviour which is disorderly according to cultural expectations. However, it can also refer to disorderly and confused thinking which is sometimes present during times of mental distress.

You will also notice that *mental health problems* or *difficulties* are referred to frequently throughout the text. These terms are more positive than 'illness'. *Problems* beg for solutions, so if we all (and this includes the client) put in some effort and keep an open mind, solutions to mental distress may be at hand. Similarly, *difficulties* suggest that effort is needed so that they are overcome.

Emotional states

Look at the faces on the opposite page. By looking closely at a person's facial expression, eyes, mouth and forehead, we can often 'read' their emotional state. Yet all the emotions shown here are part of a range of human expressions. They could belong to a mentally healthy individual or to someone experiencing mental health problems. But when someone has emotional states that are intense, prolonged or frequent, and that interfere with everyday activities or cause the individual to harm himself, herself or others, that is when we can talk about the presence of mental health difficulties.

Negative images

Perhaps you live in a city or town and have come across a person in the street who talked to himself in a loud, disturbing voice. He might have been having an argument with the 'voice' he was hearing 'inside his head'. This image of mental health distress has become familiar since shorter periods in hospital have meant that people with one of the most distressing mental health problems are now living in the community.

People who walk through the streets or stand at the bus stop shouting at no one in particular undoubtedly cause concern, fear, and other unpleasant and negative reactions in those around them. We do not like disorderly behaviour in others because most of our daily life is spent in the realm of the predictable. When something happens outside this realm, we do not understand it and feel confused or helpless – in other words out of control. It is not surprising, then, that people with severe mental health problems used to be shut away in psychiatric hospitals and asylums, so that their disorderly behaviour would not disturb the rest of the world, which, at least on the surface, appears to be ordered.

Stereotyping

Stereotyping happens when all individuals from a named group of people are ascribed a fixed image. It is safe to assume that we all do this sometimes, especially since we rarely know when we are doing it. This is because stereotyping usually occurs when our experience and knowledge of a particular group of people is limited. We have stereotypes about people based on their:

TO THINK ABOUT

You have probably heard or read about incidents of violence committed by persons who, for various reasons, have not received adequate care.

- How, in your opinion, do the media contribute to the popular view that many or most people with mental health problems are dangerous?
- What do you think are some other stereotypical views regarding people with mental health problems?
- Would you say that stereotypical descriptions express the reality concerning the majority of the clients in your care setting?

Think about each of these questions and, if you can, discuss your answers with a colleague.

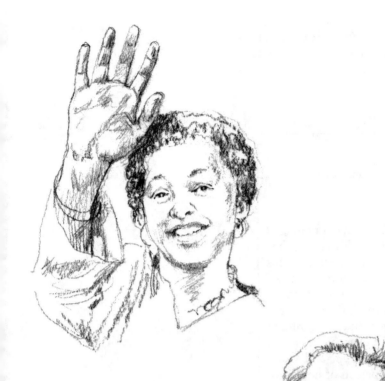

Faces say it all

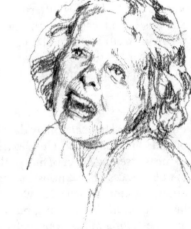

- ethnic, religious and cultural background;
- gender;
- sexual orientation;
- age;
- disabilities;
- special abilities (e.g. artistic).

If people do not know much about the effects of having mental health difficulties, or if they have never come in contact with a person with such problems, it is easy to generalise from the extreme incidents described in the newspapers. The nature of reporting is such that you are most unlikely to read about the many other people with mental health problems who are involved in professions or voluntary work, quietly attending special centres and living the best way they can like the rest of us. But as we all read about those rare incidents of aggression and violence, these characteristics soon come to represent the whole group.

ACTIVITY

Read the following case studies, then answer the questions below.

Case study A

Andrew is in his 30s and has a wife and teenage daughter. He has managed to hold on to his job as a college assistant administrator, although he has taken several long breaks from work due to the debilitating effect of his mental condition. This has been diagnosed by his GP as schizophrenia (see section 1.2). When Andrew's condition is under control, he is a reliable, conscientious and caring man. But when he is under the influence of the 'voices' which he hears inside his head, Andrew is overcome with intense fear and paranoia. On such occasions he believes that even his wife and his daughter are out to poison him or kill him in his sleep, and views everyone he meets as an enemy. Usually, after a short period of hospitalisation, Andrew is himself again, a stable and agreeable man.

Case study B

Vera is 22 and besides suffering from depression she has lost a lot of weight. She has been treated for the eating disorder anorexia nervosa and is still far from well. She is quiet, compliant and shy, with low self-esteem. She spends a lot of time on her own, usually reading, although she still manages to keep her part-time job in the local library.

Case study C

Frank is 56. There are many days each month when he cannot face stepping outside his front door. He is extremely anxious and had to retire early due to the worsening effect of his condition, which is known as agoraphobia (fear of open spaces). Being housebound, Frank enjoys housework and has learned about cooking, which he now loves. He can sometimes go out in the car with his wife on his better days, but at other times he sits in his study afraid of anyone calling at his house. His greatest fear is that he might have a panic attack so great that his heart would not be able to withstand it.

1   Having read the above examples (and also the previous *To think about* exercise), specify two ways in which each one does not fit with the stereotypical views of people with mental health problems.

2   Choose one or more clients with whom you have a good relationship and ask them to share with you their feelings about how they are viewed and treated by society because of their mental health distress.

3   List three ways in which you can contribute to creating a more positive attitude towards people with mental health difficulties.

People are individuals

Could you see in the above case studies how each of the individuals described is different? Not only do they have different kinds of mental health difficulties, but, more importantly, they are different as individuals. For example, Frank discovered his interest in cooking and taking care of the home, while Vera prefers her own company and reads a lot.

You can help your clients best by recognising them as individual human beings whose needs you, as a carer, should strive to meet. By acknowledging and building upon their strengths, you will help them to rise above their difficulties.

Help change the image

One way in which public attitudes to mental health problems can change is through awareness of what it is like to have those problems. If it is appropriate in your care setting, you, your colleagues and clients' representatives could organise some regular activities in the form of talks, perhaps with slides, given to local residents or organisations. Another way might be by recruiting volunteers from the local residents to help out during various activities in the centre or outside it. Or you might like to invite some residents to come along to your care setting for a special event, such as a celebration of the festivals of different religions, or to join in a group activity (see also Chapter 4).

It could happen to any of us

The public at large needs to be educated about mental health. If we understand that mental health is a part of everyday life, and that problems in this area of living can come up at any time for any of us, we might look upon people with mental health distress with greater understanding, imagination, compassion, and a more positive attitude.

1.2 Forms, symptoms and treatment of mental distress

How does a problem in mental health show itself?

This depends on the nature of the problem, how severe it is, how long it lasts, and many other factors including the individual's way of coping with the problem and his social support. In general, there are several ways in which a mental health problem is shown:

- *on an emotional level* – for example, frequent change of moods, feeling very low, very elated, or perhaps numb;
- *on a cognitive (or thought) level* – when concentration fails significantly or confused thinking takes over;
- *on a behavioural level* – erratic and culturally inappropriate behaviour, sometimes damaging to others (physical violence) or to himself (self-harm);
- *on a physiological level* – when someone can't sleep, for example, or is unable to eat or perform sexually.

The signs of a problem at any level are known medically as *symptoms*. This section gives the major forms of mental distress, with their symptoms and the most frequent treatments.

Depression

This is one of the most common forms of mental distress. Most of us will experience low moods and other symptoms associated with depression at some point in our lives, although the intensity and duration may not be of the kind described below.

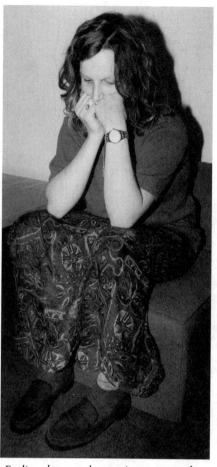

Feeling depressed sometimes means the time has come to make that difficult decision . . .

ACTIVITY

Read the following case studies, then list as many signs or symptoms of depression as you can.

Case study A

Matthew wrote in his diary:

It has been four months now since I had a good night's sleep. I keep waking up very early in the morning feeling exhausted, and a feeling of dread comes flooding in at the thought of another day which I have to live through.

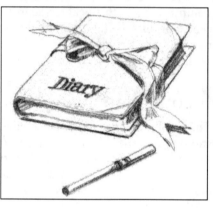

Many people from all walks of life find that keeping a diary – a personal journal – is therapeutic

I think I am worthless. Sheila (my ex-wife) has left me for another man. I know I was sexually useless for some time. My work is in a mess as well; I can no longer concentrate on what I am doing.

I have lost my appetite and I look much thinner. Although I have started to drink every day, and I am smoking a lot again, it doesn't seem to help. I have no energy for anything – even taking care of my appearance has become a huge task.

I feel that no one can help. Perhaps the only way out of this hopeless situation is to end it all.

Case study B

Sharon met her friend for lunch recently, during a time when her mood swings were stable, when no one would have guessed that she ever had any mental health problems. She told her friend how distressing it was for her to be at the mercy of these mood swings. For several months she would feel on top of the world, high and elated for no particular reason. Then, suddenly, deep depression would set in for a similar period, when she would find everything pointless and her life without any meaning. She would lose the desire to do anything and, although she would sleep a lot, she would feel exhausted. But the most frightening thing, she said, was when she had hallucinations: she experienced hearing and seeing people she knew in the past, who were not actually there. Thankfully this did not happen as often as the mood swings.

Signs or symptoms of depression

Common symptoms of depression include:

- low, depressive mood which alternates with periods of elation in what is known as manic depression;
- low self-esteem;
- poor appetite or eating more;
- sleep disturbances (not sleeping well and not for long enough, or too much sleep but still feeling tired);
- loss of sexual drive;
- lack of interest in life and lack of motivation to do things;
- delusions and hallucinations;
- feelings of guilt;
- self-neglect and neglect of one's responsibilities;
- feelings of dread and anxiety.

Forms of depression

- *Unipolar depression* (*uni* meaning one) relates to people experiencing a single depressive mood (e.g. Matthew, Case study A).
- *Bipolar* (*bi* meaning two) or *manic depression* relates to people experiencing variation between feeling very low and feeling high and elated (e.g. Sharon, Case study B).

Other terms used in the client's file

While reading your clients' files, you may come across other medical terms for depression which you do not know. It is unlikely that you will need to know the details of the client's formal diagnosis. This is there mainly for the client's doctor for whom it acts as a guide for treatment, usually for prescribing medication.

Treatment by medication

People who see their GP for depression are most likely to be prescribed anti-depressants. There are several groups of antidepressants, each consisting of a number of different medications. The major groups are:

- tricyclic and related antidepressants;
- monoamine-oxidase inhibitors (MAOIs);
- lithium salts;
- major tranquillisers.

Side effects

Different medication will have different side effects and these will vary with different people. The main effects of antidepressants are cardiac problems, blurred vision, drowsiness, urinary retention, sweating, vomiting, nausea, involuntary muscle twitching, hand tremor, diarrhoea and confusion.

ACTIVITY

1 Find out if there is a guide to medication in your care setting. If there isn't one, get in touch with MIND (see Appendix 2 for details of their central office) and ask for their *Guide to Medication*.

2 Learn about the possible side effects of the most frequently prescribed medications, such as lithium.

3 Obtain *lithium cards* (from a pharmacy) or ask a client who is prescribed lithium to show you the card.

The card explains why blood tests and other cautions are important when taking lithium.

4 Speak to your supervisor about the following:

- How would you go about finding out if your clients are experiencing any serious side effects?
- If they have serious side effects, what, if anything, should you do about it?

Treatment by ECT

ECT or *electro-convulsive therapy* involves the passing of an electric current, usually to one side of the brain. It is not understood how this treatment works, hence its use is controversial.

Stress and anxiety

Stress is the physical effect resulting from some outside experience in the form of pressure, arousal or disruption to normal functioning. If we experience prolonged stress, our body may fail to cope and our physical health may suffer. Stress can also contribute to the onset of depression and schizophrenia, and can lead to suicide.

On a physiological level, stress and anxiety have a direct effect on our central nervous system, in particular on the part whose function it is to alert our 'flight–fight' response in cases when our life is threatened. Physiological symptoms include an increase in heart rate, rapid breathing, increased perspiration and a dry mouth, raised blood sugar levels, increased blood pressure, and muscular tension and 'tension headaches'.

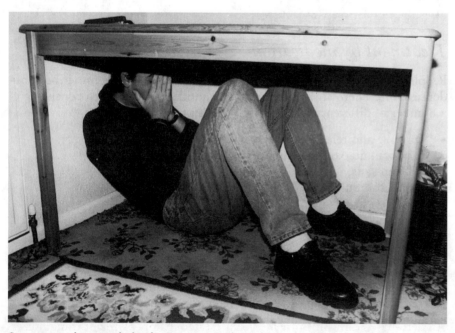

Someone with agoraphobia has an extreme fear of open spaces

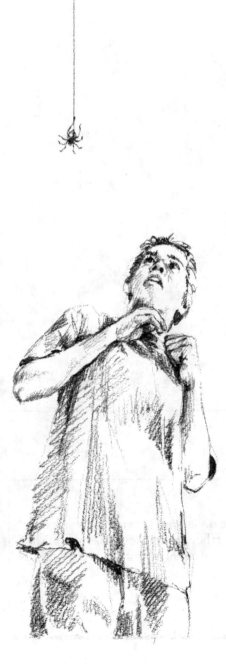

TO THINK ABOUT

What do you think your natural response would be if you feared something or someone?

Most stressful life events

On the whole there are differences among us in the way we see and experience an event. There are, nevertheless, certain events which cause similar levels of stress in all of us (see, for example, Parry *et al.*, 1981). The most stressful and damaging events are set out below in the order in which they cause stress, with the first on the list found to be most upsetting:

1 death of a spouse or a partner;
2 divorce;
3 marital separation/separation from a partner;
4 jail sentence;
5 death of a close family member;
6 injury or illness;
7 marriage;
8 losing one's job by being sacked;
9 marital reconciliation;
10 retirement.

ACTIVITY

For this activity you should try hard to be truthful about yourself, as you have to think about your most recent experiences of stress and anxiety.

1 Write down the most recent stressors (events, situations or objects, including people) that have caused you anxiety and concern.

2 Try to recall, and then write down, how you felt emotionally and physically during the time you were under stress

3 How did you cope – what did you do to help yourself during that period?

4 What would you like to do if you find yourself again in a similar situation?

Panic attacks and phobias

The physiological effects of stress and anxiety can be so overwhelming, producing the feeling of being totally out of control, and on such an intense level that people continue to live in fear of being like that again. This extremely intense anxiety may lead to what is feared – to panic attacks – so that the problem becomes circular. Panic attacks are associated with phobias, which is the name for extreme forms of fear, usually triggered by an object or situation which does not represent a real danger. Examples of phobias are:

- *agoraphobia* – fear of open spaces (the most common form);
- *claustrophobia* – fear of enclosed spaces;
- *arachnophobia* – fear of spiders.

Treatments for anxiety and phobias

Anxiety-based difficulties are medically treated mainly by major tranquillisers (for severe forms of anxiety) and MAOIs, although the treatment does not help in removing the cause. There are other medications, some of which can result in dependency on the drug (for example, benzodiazepines). Behaviour therapy (see section 1.3) has produced good results, and other therapies can be helpful. Learning to relax and using meditation and yoga can also be beneficial.

Schizophrenia

> ### CASE STUDY
>
> Ian was always a shy child who preferred his own company. In his teens, when his introversion became even greater, he showed signs of responding unemotionally to emotional situations. One day he became convinced that everyone could hear his thoughts and these were being broadcast on TV and radio. From then onwards he would avoid the media, because he was afraid of others implanting their thoughts into him by these and other means. He felt that he had no control over his thinking. Soon Ian developed delusions; one of them was his belief that he was the son of the Virgin Mary. Auditory hallucinations also appeared in the form of a 'voice' which either ridiculed him or told him to end his life.

Psychoses of schizophrenia

Psychosis is a state in which an individual cannot distinguish between reality and non-reality, such as Ian's belief that he was the son of the Virgin Mary in the above case study.

Perhaps one of the most distressing experiences of what is known as *paranoid schizophrenia* (see Case study A, page 4) is when sufferers are convinced that others, including their family, are plotting to kill them. Not surprisingly, they can become agitated and angry, while some become violent, driven by fear for their own life under the influence of the delusion.

Treatment

There is no cure for schizophrenia, but the worst symptoms can be controlled by major tranquillisers (also known as *antipsychotics*), adequate support and a social environment which is calm and free of strong emotional expression (e.g. fluctuation of anger and sadness in others).

Medical treatment has to be closely monitored by doctors to control the major symptoms and to ensure that the side effects of the drugs do not cause serious damage. Death by overdose is possible, because individuals vary in the way their body and psychological symptoms respond to the prescribed amounts of these drugs.

> ### ACTIVITY
>
> *1* Talk to your senior colleagues and ask them to tell you about two clients in your care setting who have been diagnosed as having schizophrenia.
>
> *2* Meet the clients and make an effort to get to know them as individual people, with hopes and fears, needs and aspirations.
>
> *3* When you have done this, ask yourself what effect your knowledge that they suffer from schizophrenia had on the way you related to them and on how you think of them.

Depot injections

These are also antipsychotic drugs which are injected at intervals of one to four weeks, often at the *depot clinic*. This can be a department at the hospital where the injection is given or a clinic set up at a local medical centre especially for this purpose. It is important that clients attend appointments for these injections regularly, to avoid relapse as well as adverse reactions which might occur if there is an interruption in treatment.

Other disorders

You may get to know clients who have other forms of mental health problems. For example, *obsessive–compulsive disorder* is shown by an obsession for a particular object or for frequent repetition of some behaviour. A typical example is constant hand-washing for fear of catching germs. Other disorders include *anorexia nervosa*, a condition shown when a person, usually young, stops eating for fear of getting fat, and *bulimia*, an insatiable hunger when episodes of overeating are often followed by self-induced vomiting, purging or starving.

What can you do to help during medical treatment?

Many social care mental health settings do not involve non-medically trained carers in administering the clients' medication. On the other hand, if you are expected to do this, you should do it under the strict guidance of a senior and adequately qualified worker.

Whatever the circumstances you work in, you can always help by observing any signs of serious side effects which medication might be causing.

- Always make a habit of noticing any changes in the clients which might be due to the side effects of medication. If, for example, the client develops involuntary muscle twitching, she might believe that she is becoming even more 'neurotic' when in fact this is probably due to the medication.
- Listen carefully to your clients' complaints about their physical or psychological problems. Whenever possible, check the medication they are taking and its possible side effects in a copy of *Guide to Medication* or the *British National Formulary* (ask your supervisor to keep a copy for staff use). Encourage the client to see her doctor as soon as you suspect something is wrong.
- Whenever possible, dissuade clients from eating foods which they have been advised not to because of interaction with their medication. Clients taking MAOIs should not drink alcohol or eat foods such as cheese, bananas, broad beans and yeast extract. They should also consult a *treatment card*. This can be obtained from their doctor or a pharmacist. It gives important information and instructions about taking this medication.

Yellow Cards

MIND (the mental health charity) has Yellow Cards which clients fill in, without having to give their name. Clients are asked to give information about any suspected adverse reaction to a drug they have had. This information is reported to the government drug watchdog so that the drug's safety can be improved. The Yellow Card is in the form of a leaflet: an extract is shown overleaf.

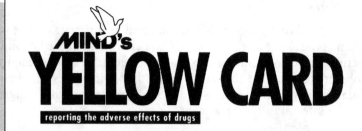

MIND's YELLOW CARD

reporting the adverse effects of drugs

Medication can be helpful in relieving symptoms of mental distress

But it can also have UNWANTED EFFECTS, sometimes extremely severe

THIS PACK IS TO HELP PEOPLE taking psychiatric medication to

REPORT unwanted effects, or adverse reactions.

MIND'S YELLOW CARD

What is an adverse drug reaction?
An adverse reaction is any bad effect or 'side' effect of a drug. For people taking psychiatric medication these may include:

- blurred vision, drowsiness, constipation

- tremor

- weight problems

- inner tension and restlessness (akathisia)

- tardive dyskinesia (a disorder of the central nervous system which involves abnormal and uncontrollable muscular movements including chewing, grimacing, lip-smacking and twitching).

The Yellow Card scheme
Doctors have a system for reporting adverse reactions to drugs, called the yellow card scheme. When patients suffer a suspected adverse reaction to a drug the doctor should complete a yellow card form and send it to the Committee on Safety of Medicines (CSM). The CSM is the body set up under the Medicines Act 1968 to advise the Secretary of State for Health on drug safety and licensing. The Yellow Card scheme, set up in 1963, is one of their major sources of information and is particularly important in identifying previously unrecognised hazards.

MIND's concerns
MIND is concerned at the massive under-reporting of adverse drug reactions. The CSM reports that only one in five doctors sends in a yellow card in any one year. The great majority of adverse reactions do not get reported at all.

MIND believes that the Committee on Safety of Medicines should receive information from the people who are actually taking medication and experiencing the side effects, or those close to them.

Extract from MIND's Yellow Card

ACTIVITY

1   Obtain a copy or batch of Yellow Cards by sending an SAE to:

MIND Publications Y/C
15–19 Broadway
London E15 4BQ

2   With your supervisor's permission, arrange to have a discussion with clients about promoting the use of these cards, taking note of the concerns they express.

ACTIVITY

1 Name, if you can, some advantages of the medical model's approach to mental health problems. (You might find a clue in the term 'illness'.)

2 Write down two examples of its disadvantages.

Positive aspects of the medical view of mental distress

When someone who feels unhappy, guilty and very dissatisfied with her life is finally told that she suffers from a depressive illness, she might experience relief. This is because having a medical term helps to lift self-blame and the feeling of being personally inadequate which might be implied when a non-biological, emotional basis for the mental distress is given. Secondly, medical diagnosis suggests that there is an easy solution: the client is now a patient who simply follows the doctor's orders. To do this is easier than to confront and examine your life in the process of psychotherapy, for example. However, the passive role of the patient, although easier to fulfil, has the disadvantage that goes with stripping someone of the individual strengths and resources which are needed to deal with the mental distress. Another major disadvantage is that of side effects, which can include dependency on the drugs used.

Use of language – labelling

Categories of mental distress exist mainly as a guide to monitor signs or symptoms and for doctors to prescribe medication.

You will be encouraged throughout this book to relate to your clients as individuals, and therefore you should be aware of the unhelpful and more damaging aspects of diagnostic labelling. One instance of this is when such labels are used in a context other than medical to describe individuals.

There is a fine but important line between calling someone a 'schizophrenic' and saying that he has been diagnosed as suffering from 'schizophrenia'. In the first instance, there is an implied suggestion that the label 'schizophrenic' refers to the whole person. This has the effect of depersonalisation, stripping the individual of all characteristics that make him human.

Labelling people according to some unpleasant and socially undesirable characteristics – as mental disorder is considered to be – and then using the label in a wide range of contexts can have the effect of permanently attaching the negative symptoms to people who have been diagnosed. This can make it more difficult for them to fight to free themselves from their problems. In your day-to-day contact with clients, strive to see them and relate to them as people and as individuals. Only in your communication with other professionals is it fully justifiable to use the name given to their mental health problem.

Further reading

Some useful leaflets and booklets on different forms of mental health problems and their treatment can be obtained free from MIND (see Appendix 2 for the central office address; use this to get details of regional offices in England and Wales and information and help on a wide range of mental health problems).

Other helpful publications include:

★ Cooper, C. 1988: *Living with Stress*. Penguin.
★ Wren, J. 1992: *Managing Anxiety* (2nd edition). Pepar.
★ Hurst, V. R. 1986: *Agoraphobia*. Faber and Faber. This is written by a woman who suffered from agoraphobia and, after many years, found the help she needed. It is an interesting and balanced account, with useful information.

For your information

★ *The National Schizophrenia Fellowship* provides information (including a booklet about schizophrenia written from the medical perspective) for workers and clients. You can obtain details from 28 Castle Street, Kingston-upon-Thames, Surrey KT1 1SS. Tel. 0181 547 3937.

★ *Hearing Voices Network* has local groups in England, Scotland and Wales. It can supply a free copy of *Voices* magazine, featuring stories, letters and poems on the subject of hearing and coping with voices by clients, as well as other publications on the subject. The national office can be contacted for more details: Hearing Voices Network, c/o Creative Support, Fourways House, 15 Tariff Street, Manchester M1 2EP. Tel. 0161 228 3896.

1.3 Models of mental distress and talking treatments

There are more than half a dozen major models of mental distress. Each one is both a theory about the causes and a set of treatments or therapies. Each model has its own set of concepts and language related to those concepts. Generally, there are two distinct kinds of models: medical, with a biological basis for mental disorders; and psychological, with psycho-social explanations.

The major models and the people associated with them are presented in the table below. Approaches that are often used together are placed in the same box: cognitive and behavioural models, for example, where cognitive–behavioural therapy uses concepts and skills derived from both models.

Models and their therapies

Model	Causes	Treatment	Concepts
Psychoanalytic (Freud, Jung, Adler, Klein)	conflict between id, ego and superego, repression	psychoanalytic therapy – introspection, interpretation	id, ego, superego, the unconscious, defence mechanism
Medical (orthodox psychiatry; Kraepelin, Bleuler)	biochemical, genetic, organic	medication, ECT, psycho-surgery	illness, symptoms, diagnosis, treatment
Cognitive (Beck, Ellis)	irrational beliefs and thoughts	cognitive therapy	faulty automatic thinking
Behavioural (Watson, Pavlov, Skinner)	learned maladaptive behaviour	behaviour therapy	behaviour modification
Existential (Kierkegaard, Sartre)	existential anxiety	existential therapy	angst (anxiety), freedom, creativity
Humanistic (Maslow, Rogers)	self-denial	client-centred therapy	authenticity, self-actualisation

The above table is only a rough outline of what the major models represent; there are other variations and theoretical approaches, which adopt ideas from

TO THINK ABOUT

1 Why do you think we have so many models in mental health?

2 Which of the above models have you heard of being used in your care setting?

the major models, but also add something new. Examples of these are transactional analysis (TA), gestalt therapy, family therapy, and integrative therapy. The suggested reading at the end of this section shows where you can get more detailed descriptions of models and therapies.

No single explanation is perfect

Perhaps your instinct tells you that we would not have so many different theories and ways of dealing with mental health difficulties if there were a single approach which would have all the answers, not only regarding the causes but, more importantly, the treatments and cures. The complexity of human nature makes the area of mental health one of the most challenging for scientists. Many models could be viewed in a positive manner, not as opposing each other but as complementary or as alternative approaches to suit individual preference.

This is a very large subject and here we can only give an outline of the most frequently used talking therapies. These are derived from the models outlined in the previous table and focus on specific aspects which you may find helpful to consider as you work with clients.

Talking treatments

These are psychologically based therapies which were developed using the concepts and theoretical base of different models, such as those given in the previous table.

- *Psychotherapy* (or just *therapy,* as in *cognitive therapy*) is a form of talking therapy which usually engages a client (or clients for group therapy) over some time, for example one or two years or more. It aims at making fundamental personality changes, so that the individual relates to himself or herself and others in a more helpful way.
- *Counselling* is more problem oriented. For example, bereavement counselling aims to help clients through their grieving process (see section 5.3). It usually lasts for a shorter period than therapy.

Cognitive therapy

If you have a good rapport with the clients in your care setting, you may get to know how they really feel and think about themselves and life in general. This may lead you to discover that they tend to engage in negative and self-defeating thinking. This is particularly so of depressed people who, according to Beck, have

- a negative view of themselves;
- a negative view of the world;
- a negative view of the future.

The aim of therapy is to change the client's pattern of negative thinking, because positive and more constructive thoughts give rise to positive emotions. Other cognitive therapists, such as Ellis, believe that the causes of mental disorder and unhappiness originate in our false, irrational beliefs; for example, that everyone must like us, or that the world is or must be a just place to live in.

A cognitive therapist or counsellor challenges the client's irrational beliefs and unhelpful thinking, and often prescribes him tasks such as writing down his negative thoughts about himself and replacing them with positive ones, in order to help him adopt more constructive beliefs and thoughts. It is hoped this will lead to more constructive behaviour and actions.

ACTIVITY

Choose two clients in your care setting who suffer from modest to severe depression (their files will give the information you need). Over a period of several days, listen to their conversations with other clients and with care workers. Then make notes as you focus on:

- how they feel and think about themselves;
- their feelings and thoughts about the world at large;
- their attitude towards the future – are they pessimistic or optimistic?

A note of caution for care workers

The influence of the cognitive therapy approach is found in all areas of life where negative attitudes or patterns of behaviour may be an obstacle to satisfying living and working. 'Be positive!', 'Think positively!', and similar phrases are part of everyday life. These phrases can give encouragement and increase optimism when used appropriately. But you should be careful not to use such phrases whenever the client appears to slip into a negative frame of mind, especially when she wants to tell you about her distressing emotions and thoughts or give you an account of an upsetting experience. A client who is not allowed to share her feelings of, for example, hurt, rejection, isolation or fear, but who is expected always to 'be positive', will feel even more isolated and rejected (and so more depressed) because of the implied message that she should not be herself.

> **TO THINK ABOUT**
>
> The cognitive model adopts a motto from the philosopher Epictetus (first century AD), which claims that we are not disturbed by things but by our view of them. Can you think of situations or examples when this might be true?

Behaviour therapy

Behaviour therapy uses methods of treating an individual's unhelpful behaviour. Such methods are based on theories which explain the different ways in which we learn. One way of learning is known as *classical conditioning*, which represents learning by association. For example, if as a driver you have been in a car crash, you might have experienced a panic attack because of fear (see section 1.2). Your future response might be such that merely being in a car will bring on a panic attack.

Unlearning this unhelpful behaviour which prevents you from driving might then be undertaken by, for example, learning a new, positive association with driving a car. This will eventually replace the upsetting association of the panic attack. For instance, you could be taught a relaxation technique such as imagining your sense of achievement when arriving in your car for an important appointment. The new learning is often taken in small steps, at the client's pace: for example, first learning to relax in a stationary car, then sitting in a car that is moving a short distance, then a longer distance, and finally being in the driver's seat yourself. This particular method is called *systematic desensitisation*.

Other methods used by a behaviour therapist might include a suggestion that the client gives herself some reward whenever she succeeds in staying away from unhelpful behaviour, such as going for a day without a cigarette. This is based on the notion that, especially when we are young, we learn behaviour by receiving rewards, punishments or indifference from those around us.

How to deal with unhelpful behaviour in your work

In your work with clients you might choose, for example, to ignore behaviour which the client displays just to attract attention, such as shouting and demanding something from you rather than waiting her turn. This does not mean that behaviour which is upsetting to other people, such as showing a racist or sexist attitude, should be ignored and allowed to go unchallenged.

Use of behaviour therapy

Behaviour therapy is particularly successful in helping people to overcome anxiety, phobias and obsessive–compulsive behaviours (see section 1.2). In conjunction with cognitive therapy, it is also used to help depression.

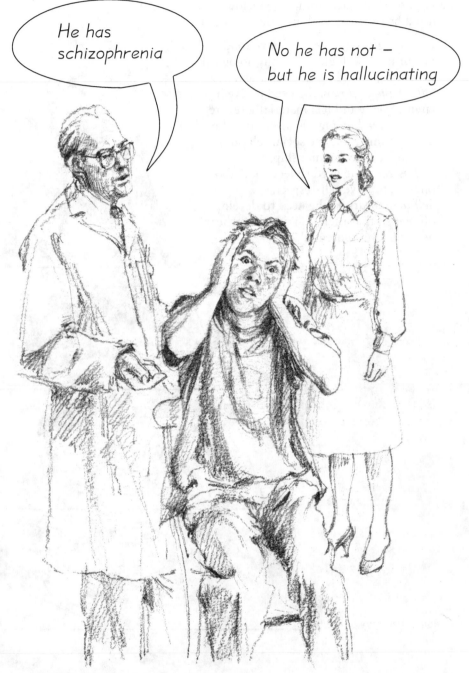

Medical model versus behavioural model

Client-centred therapy

The client-centred approach to counselling and psychotherapy derives from the humanistic model (see table on page 14). The word 'humanistic' suggests that this approach forces us to think what being human really means in terms of our needs and aspirations.

What clients might need

The needs of your clients – whether practical, emotional or educational – are bound to be included in Maslow's humanistic *hierarchy of needs*. These

the 'needs' which, according to Maslow, we all have. They are listed below in ascending order of importance:

1 *Physiological*: the need to have food and to perform all biological and physiological functions, including sleep and sex.
2 *Safety and security*: the need to live in a safe environment and feel materially secure.
3 *Love and belonging*: the need to feel part of a community, to have social relationships and to have companionship.
4 *Self-esteem*: the need to feel good about oneself, to have self-respect.
5 *Self-actualisation*: the need to develop oneself so that each individual reaches her or his full potential.

Maslow's hierarchy of needs

How it can be used

Client-centred therapy or counselling is reflected in the way in which the helper communicates with the client. For instance, when asked for your advice or opinion about something, instead of giving the answer, you pose the same question back to the client. You are thus forcing him to think for himself and to make his own decisions. This is why this way of working is often referred to as a *non-directive* approach – the client will not be told by the helper what to do. This can give a feeling of self-determination to the client, who might previously have been treated as a helpless victim or vulnerable patient. The implied message is that you see him as a person capable of thinking for himself, knowing best his own needs and abilities.

Uses and abuses of non-directive communication

You should be careful not to overdo this kind of talk with clients, because it can give the impression that you do not wish to be helpful or to share your views. For example, people from some ethnic communities who might expect a professional to give them direction and practical help could interpret your response as unhelpful.

Family therapy

Family therapy is becoming an increasingly popular talking treatment. Its approach is distinct from other treatments because its central belief is that the mental distress of one individual is not a problem of that person alone, but one of the whole family. The family is viewed as a *system* which, like any other, has its particular way of working.

The job of a family therapist is to find out by observation and listening how the client's family system works – that is, how its members interact and relate to each other – because that will give clues about how the problems are maintained.

Ethnic projects

In the UK there are now care settings, sometimes known as *projects* (which, unfortunately, can indicate that they are funded for only a limited time), for people of various ethnic and racial origins who, beside the Western approaches to mental health, might also employ some other approach. For example, some Afro-Caribbean people are influenced by the *theory of emotion*, which describes mental and some physical disorders as stemming from an excess of emotions such as anger, jealousy and hatred. Others, such as the Unity Centre for Black people in South London, adopt a practice of Christian faith using prayer and meditation as a way to holistic healing, while also accepting the traditional medicine of orthodox psychiatry. Further details are supplied in Appendix 2.

Avoid making assumptions

While you should try to find out, be aware of and respect other beliefs and practices which people from different ethnic and cultural backgrounds favour, it is important that you do not make false assumptions. For example, the theory of emotion has followers among White Westerners as well. The difference seems to be that the Western professionals are more influenced by the orthodox psychiatry on which they depend for funding and consequently for their employment. This makes it more difficult for them to apply holistic methods to already existing orthodox care settings.

Non-medical perspectives

The psychological talking treatments presented so far do not strictly prevent the use of medical treatments as well. This is because professionals who practise counselling and psychotherapy by and large see some value in the use of drugs, or the use of the Mental Health Act 1983 (see section 1.5). However, there are professionals and clients who totally disagree with any use of medication and anything which stems from the medical perspective – including legislation to enforce treatment – believing this to be inappropriate, unhelpful and damaging to clients and society.

I have placed these views under the title 'non-medical', although anti-medical might be more appropriate.

Although not quite the same, these views have influenced and are similar to the *existential* model, according to which mental health distress is a part of everyday living where all of us have to deal with anxieties *(angst)* and sometimes crises, which are part of human existence.

The origins

Most current anti-medical philosophies and practices began in the *anti-psychiatry* movement of the 1960s and 1970s.

R. D. Laing in the UK and T. Szasz in the USA were the main supporters of a belief that the medical treatment of people with mental distress was serving those powerful sections of society whose interest was to subdue and control less powerful individuals. These were mainly people from the lower classes, women, ethnic minority groups, and individuals whose nonconformist behaviour threatened those in power.

According to this movement, a possible alternative explanation for mental distress was that a client might be someone who as a child disobeyed his parents and later defies cultural behaviours that represent the social norm. As Laing puts it, from being 'good' (obedient), the child becomes 'bad' (disobedient) and then 'mad', as he is labelled by the medical model and society.

Current influences

The anti-psychiatry perspective, presented in language easily understood by lay people, continues to inspire some workers in mental health but also people who have had adverse experience of medical treatment and the psychiatric system. However, only workers who do not depend on public funds or government grants can afford to be followers of such views. Some advocacy groups (see section 3.8) whose funding is independent and uncertain are influenced by the anti-psychiatry movement.

Szasz, who continues to influence the existential movement, questions the value of therapy because it relies on communication taking place between a client and a therapist who are not equal. So the more powerful of the two, the therapist, can influence the client's value system – which poses ethical questions.

Self-help groups

These are various groups of people formed by individuals who have the same kind of problem (for example, depression, agoraphobia or alcohol abuse). The members, one or more of whom might have overcome the problem, encourage and support each other.

What helps best?

This depends very much on the individual. A particular talking treatment may suit one person better than another, because people are different – just as a medical treatment might help some people but not others. In the same way, counselling or psychotherapy is not appropriate treatment for everybody.

Holistic help – such as acupuncture and homoeopathy – is being used more commonly, and self-help group support also plays an important part for many people with mental distress.

TO THINK ABOUT

1 Can communication between individuals exist without some mutual or one-sided influence in opinion, feeling, thinking or information gathering?

2 Think about individuals in your life who had the most influence on you. Who are they? Why do you think you were influenced by them?

ACTIVITY

1 Talk to your senior colleagues. Ask them which approach to mental health treatment they favour, and why.

2 If you were having a serious mental health problem such as severe depression, what treatment would you like to have? Why?

The general picture

The causes of mental distress remain undetermined, apart from a few conditions such as depression during the menopause due to hormonal imbalance.

Persistent use of the term 'illness', as in 'mental illness', contributes greatly to the general public's view that the causes of mental distress are biological in origin. This is because the medical model is the oldest, has the most respect and therefore carries more authority. It also attracts much more funding than other approaches and adds to the wealth of the pharmaceutical companies. But it does more than this: the medical model could be said to 'save the face' of the client, a family and society at large, by removing responsibility from them.

Other non-medical psycho-sociologically based approaches tend to do the opposite. They attribute causes to the environment, be it poor economic conditions (stress over lack of work, housing, diet) or social conditions, as in the way some families interact with one another or some parents use their mental and psychological power against their children. It is easy to see why the most radical person among those supporting the non-medical approaches, R. D. Laing, has been exiled by his psychiatrist colleagues and others in power. His views represent a threat to the present social and political order. This is quite understandable: no one likes to be told that they have been totally wrong in fundamental things such as bringing up and educating children, or not treating each other with enough honesty, compassion and humility.

As a society we need courage if we are ever to succeed in finding the real cause and cure for mental distress. For this to happen, we might perhaps start by giving an equal chance to all or most of the existing models and their therapies. In some ways this is already happening with other approaches, and holistic medicine is becoming the first choice for some clients. So far, however, these treatments are mostly for those who can afford to pay.

Further reading

Making Sense of Treatments and *Understanding Talking Treatments* are written and published by MIND for lay people. You should be able to obtain them free from MIND (see Appendix 2 for details).

Other books which you may find useful include:

★ Burnard, P. 1992: *What is Counselling? A Personal and Practical Guide.* Gale Centre Publications.
★ Eagan, G. 1986: *The Skilled Helper* (3rd edition). Brooks Cole.
★ Herbert, M. 1986: *Psychology for Social Workers.* Macmillan.
★ Laing, R. D. 1963: *Sanity, Madness and the Family.* Penguin.
★ Laing, R. D. 1969: *The Divided Self.* Penguin.
★ Nelson-Jones, R. 1993: *You can Help.* Cassell.

If you wish to learn more about how to apply the different therapies outlined in this section, especially if you aim to take higher qualifications, there is a readable series of slim paperbacks, the *Counselling in Action* series published by Sage, with titles such as *Cognitive–Behaviour Counselling in Action* and *Existential Counselling in Practice*.

1.4 Community care: legislation and language

What is community care?

If we were suffering from some kind of long-term mental health problems or other health failure which did not demand hospital care, most of us would prefer to stay at home with family and friends. In the White Paper *Caring for People: Community Care in the Next Decade and Beyond* (1989), the government recognised a need for a greater commitment in the 1990s to improve community-based services for health and social care. It proposed changes to develop high-quality local services which would be in line with national policies.

The main aims of the changes are to help people to:

- live in a homely environment in the community or in their own homes with the support of day care (for some therapeutic purposes), domiciliary care (help in running the home), primary health care, and other appropriate forms of support;
- develop their full potential by helping them to relearn the skills of independent living;
- have a greater choice in how they want to live and what services they want to use.

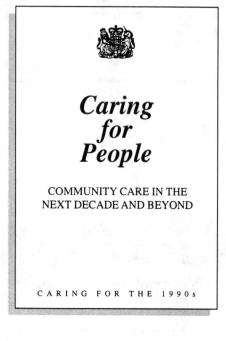

Caring for People

COMMUNITY CARE IN THE NEXT DECADE AND BEYOND

CARING FOR THE 1990s

The National Health Service and Community Care Act 1990

This Act put forward changes which are to be implemented so that local health authorities, social services departments, and independent agencies in the private and voluntary sectors contribute in the most effective way to caring for people in the community. One of the major changes is that local authorities should play a key role and have a major responsibility (in collaboration with medical and other relevant professionals) for assessing the clients' needs, designing care plans and arranging services for clients. Social services staff are no longer expected to be the main providers of care, but are responsible for organising and co-ordinating care. Their most important contribution is that of taking on the role of 'case manager' for individual clients. This may involve arranging assessment (e.g. for housing), choosing the appropriate form of care, making sure the resources are used most effectively, and similar tasks. You will find more about the case management approach to care in Chapter 3.

The specific nature of changes, and especially who does what, will depend on the care setting – some may have to undergo greater changes than others.

ACTIVITY

1 Ask your colleagues or your supervisor to explain to you the most significant changes which have occurred recently, or are soon to take place, as a direct result of government policies such as the National Health Services and Community Care Act.

2 Can you (or can they) see how these changes will improve caring for clients in the community?

Greater flexibility

Generally speaking, the changes demand that carers be more flexible and learn new skills. For example, the old division between health care and social care is sometimes blurred. For instance, a psychiatric nurse might also be given the role of case manager. Collaboration and multi-agency work is also encouraged. Local authorities are responsible for holding the budget allocated by the government and using it in a cost-effective manner. They contract other agencies who offer care and take on the role of the main *purchaser of care*. Their negotiation for the best offers of care with a wider range of providers should encourage competition among them, thus creating incentives for expansion and development, especially in the independent sector. The result of this should be that clients will benefit because they now have a greater choice of service.

Supervision registers

Mental health and social care, as well as community care practices, are presently undergoing rapid changes with more input from the government. An important policy implemented by the Secretary of Health from 1995 is that of *supervision registers*. All mental health care agencies have to keep a special register containing confidential medical information for people with severe mental distress in their locality. Such information will be available to all relevant care professionals so that they can check if a client who comes to them is already on a register and therefore being 'supervised' (in terms of their treatment and care) somewhere else.

Supervised discharge orders and aftercare under supervision

The Mental Health (Patients in the Community) Act 1995, a controversial piece of legislation, came into effect in April 1996. It concerns people who are due to leave psychiatric hospitals, especially after enforced hospitalisation (see section 1.5), who have been assessed as falling into the 'high risk' category – those who suffer severe mental distress and have a record of not complying with treatment programmes. A condition for their discharge from the hospital will demand their consent to being 'supervised' in their life in the community. This requires that they submit to advice about where and what kind of treatment they will receive, and where they will live, work or go for training. The aim is to ensure that people at risk do not lose contact with mental health services and so become a risk to others or to themselves. If a person does not co-operate with such 'orders', he could be reassessed for readmission.

The objection of some professionals to this legislation is that it will put off clients from seeking help, especially from social workers who will play a major role and who might be viewed as policing agents rather than carers.

Potential problems

The notion that the registers and supervision discharge orders are used to keep an eye on some clients, suggesting policing, might contribute to the negative image of people with mental health problems – implying that they are irresponsible and perhaps even violent, so must be watched. Some professionals will be put in a difficult position, because if clients view care workers as administrators of the law with the power to restrict their personal freedom, they will lose trust in them and avoid seeking help.

Potential advantages

If an individual wants care workers in various settings to know of him in case he has a relapse during which he might become disoriented, confused and forgetful, the register could be valuable. The client can then be sure that, if he experiences crises due to a relapse, he will be picked up by the profes-

---

ACTIVITY

1 Write down your thoughts on how a client would be helped by having his or her personal details displayed in special supervision registers.

2 Give examples of situations in which highly confidential information regarding clients whose names are on the register could be misused.

TO THINK ABOUT

1 Do you think that a policy such as the implementation of supervised discharge orders, which implies a tight control of people with severe mental distress, contributes to the public image of mental health clients? If so, how?

2 How do you think this policy might affect clients?

sionals wherever he happens to find himself. When appropriate, he will be directed to those who are responsible for managing his care. For example, he could be reminded that he needs to visit his doctor to receive his ongoing medical treatment.

Supervised discharge orders could have a similar benefit if the client truly co-operates. Yet co-operation is difficult when you don't have a choice.

Care versus coercion

The problem is, however, that once something becomes law, clients could be pressurised to 'agree' to be supervised on discharge from hospitals, because if they do not their hospitalisation might be prolonged – or at least they might fear that this will happen, which has the same effect. Care given by a professional who is a 'supervisor' to clients adds to the clients' stress and anxiety, and so its effectiveness may well be jeopardised.

Professional and moral dilemmas

Problems such as these show how easily mental health care may become a battlefield of professional and moral dilemmas. They also demonstrate how difficult it can be to achieve goals of community care: to ensure that clients are cared for and receive their treatment while living in the community, on the one hand, and enjoy personal freedom (and the self-respect which comes with it) and a choice of care, on the other.

Other legislation
Residential care

Residential homes have to be registered under the Registered Homes Act 1984. This is to ensure that the premises are suitable and meet set standards of facilities and services. The health authority registers and inspects nursing homes; social services authorities do the same for care homes. Care homes run by social services also have to be inspected, under a provision of the Community Care Act 1990.

The Wagner Report 1988 is also relevant to residential care. It contains many recommendations which have been incorporated into other legislation that has influenced the work of social services in this area.

Patient's Charter

Discussions are now taking place regarding the improvement of care in the community for people with mental distress under the *Patient's Charter*. For example, every individual in need of services will be entitled to be assessed for a care plan for his or her individual care. This means that more resources will be available.

The Carers Recognition and Services Act 1995

According to this Act, from April 1996, local authorities have to assess not only the clients' needs but also those of their carers. This will be particularly relevant in circumstances where, for example, disabled clients are cared for by family members or someone else. Disability includes severe mental distress which necessitates some form of help by others.

A growing concern that some young children are carers should alert mental health professionals, especially when assessing care needs within single parent families, to be aware of a child who might play the major role of a carer and who is unlikely to know where to turn for help – which must be delivered according to this Act.

What you need to know

In the course of your work you will come across other legislation and hear about the policies of your own or other care agencies. Some of these laws, such as the Health and Safety Act and Health and Safety at Work Act 1974, will be of direct relevance to your work and to the way in which you provide care. When appropriate in this workbook, this legislation will be referred to in relation to the work you do. You may also hear about other legislation which will be of greater concern for your employer or more senior colleagues. You do not need to learn about every piece of legislation which is connected with your work: you are not a law student. However, you should know how to find out more if such information is going to be directly relevant to your work with clients and to your own individual rights and responsibilities as a care worker.

New language in community care

With the latest legislation and the resultant changes, new terms are being used to describe the new forms of care being given and the government's new attitudes to care. The meaning of some of these terms is set out below.

- *Provider of care*: any agency which provides some form of care.
- *Purchaser of care*: the agency with whose budget the care is being provided. Usually it will be the local social services or the health authority.
- *Packages of care*: services designed for clients after their needs and the needs of their carers have been assessed.
- *Case (or care) manager*: a social worker, nurse or other professional responsible for overall management and co-ordination of the care given to an individual (see also Chapter 3).
- *Consumer*: a client who uses services.
- *Community care plan*: a plan which local authorities have to prepare and review annually, describing how they intend to achieve their objectives and fulfil their role in accordance with government policies, especially the Community Care Act. Health authorities have to produce a *health plan*.
- *Supervision register*: confidential records of clients with severe mental health problems linked by computer between services, designed to keep such clients in touch with the services they need most.

Mind your language

Specific terms used in a particular profession become part of language. This is often spoken of as *professional jargon*. Ordinary words and phrases have special meanings and can be used as a more direct way of communicating with those who also know and use the same language.

In a multi-disciplinary team, or in collaborative work involving carers from different fields, levels and kinds of training, workers do not always realise that the terms they employ may create a barrier between them and others with different specialisations. If you find yourself in situations where

---

ACTIVITY

1 Listen to the language that your senior colleagues use while talking about their work with clients and legislation. Jot down (unobtrusively) any words or phrases which you do not understand.

2 Find an opportunity to ask your colleagues to explain the meaning of these terms and the legislation to which they relate. Meeting with your supervisor might provide an opportunity for this.

the use of too much professional language gets in the way of communicating and caring more effectively, talk to your colleagues or your supervisor. If you do so, you will probably soon find that you are also speaking for others in your team.

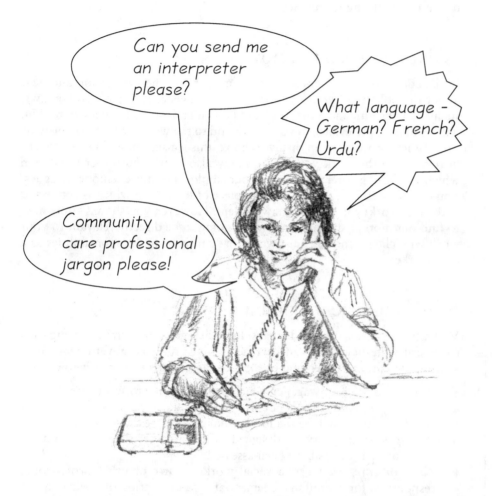

1.5 The Mental Health Act 1983

Why do we have legislation in mental health care?

Consider a person who has a severe physical illness yet refuses to go to a doctor or into hospital to receive treatment. If this individual is left free she will be a 'danger to herself' because her physical health will deteriorate so much that her life might be in danger. Consider also that disability caused by this illness makes it extremely difficult for the patient's family or other carers to cope. This suggests that the untreated condition of the sufferer might represent 'a danger to others'. For example, during the course of caring for the patient who has become disabled due to her refusal of treatment, the carer may suffer back injury as well as psychological strain and stress.

We may continue to speculate about such a patient and suggest that by refusing treatment she deliberately allows her health to become worse, and that such self-inflicted ill health, which may lead to permanent disability, even death, is not by its outcome very different from self-harm inflicted by a person with mental distress.

We do not have legislation to enforce hospitalisation and treatment of a person who refuses professional help when suffering physical illness. Yet, if the same person experiences mental distress and refuses treatment which, according to professionals, will prevent her mental health becoming worse or her being a danger to herself or others, she will be detained and treated against her wishes under the provisions of the Mental Health Act 1983.

Mental health is more unpredictable

We do not know a lot about the causes and cures of mental distress, although we have 'educated guesses' about the causes and a range of treatments which many sufferers find helpful. This suggests that there is more mystery surrounding mental health than physical health. But the important difference between the two is that the behaviours and moods displayed by a person with mental health problems are more unpredictable, and can get out of control. This makes it natural for those around such a person to be concerned and afraid, both for their own safety and for the safety of the sufferer. However, only a very small percentage of people with mental health problems are dangerous. The Mental Health Act 1983 exists for them – to help them and to protect the public. Yet, like some other imperfect solutions to problems concerning the health and safety of individuals within a society, it may at times fail.

When is it appropriate to apply the Mental Health Act?

Laws are the legal outcomes of political forces working within a society. They are made by the more powerful sections of that society who can choose either to include or to exclude the wishes and interests of the less powerful members. Sometimes the difficulty of ensuring that a particular law is helpful (or 'just') lies in its interpretation and application. The question therefore for many professionals might not be *why* we have the Mental Health Act, but *when* it is appropriate to apply it. Their job is to arrive at a decision that will be right for everyone who will be affected by it, including or especially the client, in each individual circumstance. This is not always easy: individuals' experience of mental distress can vary greatly, which makes it difficult to make predictions about a person's danger to herself or others.

What is the Mental Health Act 1983?

The Act is a piece of legislation which clarifies the nature of the powers and the roles that various professionals and others, such as the clients' closest relatives, have in relation to individuals experiencing mental health difficulties under specified conditions. These conditions are that:

- the client is suffering from a mental disorder (although the Act also makes some provisions for people with learning difficulties);
- the nature or the severity of an individual's mental distress necessitates professional intervention such as compulsory detention and/or medical treatment without which his or her mental health may get worse;
- without intervention the individual is a danger to himself or herself (for example, by self-harm or through self-neglect);
- the individual represents a danger to others.

Not all these conditions need to exist for the Act to be applied. The first one, that the individual suffers mental distress, plus any other condition listed above can be sufficient.

Applications of the Act

The Act plays an especially important role in the life of psychiatric wards and psychiatric hospitals. Any person, regardless of whether she or he lives in a residential home, a hostel, own home, or is homeless can, during personal crises (and without previous history of mental health difficulties) and/or during extreme mental distress, become subject to the provisions of the Act. This may mean compulsory hospitalisation, compulsory medical treatment, or both.

A brief outline of the Act

The Mental Health Act 1983 consists of ten parts which contain provisions about the following issues:

- compulsory admission to hospital and guardianship and the rights and roles of detained clients and their relatives;
- hospitalisation and guardianship of those who have committed a crime and are suffering from mental health problems;
- powers and roles of professionals, especially approved social workers, doctors and hospital managers;
- powers of mental health review tribunals;
- moving clients within different parts of the UK and dealing with clients from abroad;
- looking after detained persons' affairs and their property.

The Act also describes the role of the Secretary of State. When appropriate it makes references to different parts of the UK – Scotland, Wales and the Channel Islands.

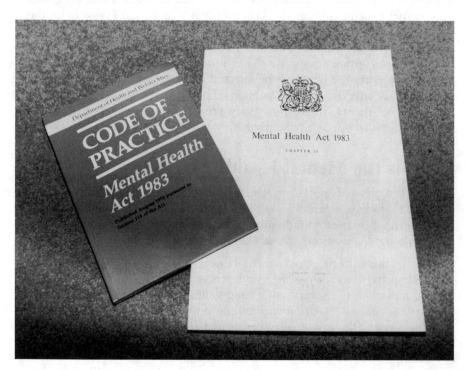

What you need to know

Many *sections* of the Act and their application are not appropriate for this workbook. Some of your senior colleagues, such as *approved social workers*, are trained to take on important responsibilities in relation to administering the Act, but you will not be expected to have such a role. However, if your client wishes to tell you about his or her recent experience of being *sectioned* – the term used for detention under different sections of the Act – having some knowledge of the Act would be useful. By reading the case study below you will get some idea of how and when this legislation might be applied.

Social work training and the Act

If you are having social work training (such as CQSW), you should read a much fuller description of the Mental Health Act 1983, preferably the Act itself and the *Code of Practice*, which gives a clear explanation of how to apply its various provisions. Details of these publications are given at the end of this chapter.

CASE STUDY

Paula's parents were beside themselves. They did not know how to cope with their daughter's sudden turns in moods and behaviour. Although she had never been very communicative, Paula had never experienced mental health difficulties until the news that she failed her first year's exams, for which she seemed to blame her parents and so turned against them. Paula became very argumentative, even abusive towards her parents. From that day on her moods changed frequently from sadness and dejection to anger, while at other times an unexpected good humour would take over accompanied by laughter, singing, and dancing. Her carelessness during this time caused many accidents around the house, such as broken and damaged objects. Her parents could not recognise their daughter and began to fear that her behaviour would cause serious harm to them or to herself. After two weeks of trying to cope with her they admitted that she and they needed outside help.

The family doctor was consulted. In his presence Paula expressed an uncontrollable euphoric behaviour (shown by her extremely high-spirited mood as she laughed inappropriately) and during it had a nasty fall injuring her leg. Her parents agreed with the doctor that their daughter should be hospitalised in order to be properly assessed and, if necessary, given treatment. But Paula was not in a mood to listen to any reasonable discussion and could not be persuaded to agree to a voluntary hospitalisation. Her GP then arranged an ambulance and Paula was detained in the hospital under Section 2 of the Mental Health Act 1983 (outlined on the next page).

Section 2 of the Act: Compulsory admission for assessment

The reasons for Paula's admission under this provision of the Act were that she suffered mental health problems which were sufficiently severe to warrant hospitalisation, and that she was a danger to herself (her fall during her uncontrollable euphoria showed this) and possibly to others. Her parents feared that she might harm them, although there was no evidence for this. Only one of the final two conditions is necessary for detention under Section 2. As the nature of her mental distress was not known, she needed to be assessed.

In Paula's example her parents made an application for her to be hospitalised, but this can also be done by other relatives or by an approved social worker. However, an application for admission can only be successful if it is signed by two registered doctors, who must give their independent medical recommendations for compulsory hospital admission for assessment. Paula's GP provided one signature and this is the preferable arrangement. Detention under Section 2 can last up to 28 days.

If Paula lived alone, and her parents did not know of her hospitalisation, the approved social worker who co-ordinates admission would have been under a statutory obligation to inform them (or her other nearest relative) about detention, whenever possible.

The experience of being sectioned

People who have gone through this experience often have a range of negative feelings about the powers which some professionals have over them. If you did the previous activity, you may have identified with a client who felt powerless, angry, afraid or terrified, confused, disoriented, humiliated, misunderstood and victimised, and who, as a result, mistrusted the professionals or relatives who began the compulsory detention. You may wonder how helpful, in the long-term, is a treatment which – although it may work as a short-term measure to control some symptoms – is given to clients who have these negative feelings towards care provided under such circumstances.

However, some clients might express positive feelings about compulsory detention and treatment later, when discharged from the hospital, because they genuinely recognise and fear their symptoms of mental distress which they cannot control. Others might claim positive attitudes towards their detention and treatment as a way of more quickly achieving discharge from the hospital by telling professionals what they think they want to hear. Thus they may act like a prisoner who gets discharged sooner because of 'good behaviour'. This is one of the major concerns about enforcing supervised discharge registers or similar legislation (discussed in section 1.4).

A right to appeal against compulsory detention

A person who believes that he or she has been detained by the Act unjustly or mistakenly has a right to appeal for 'an order for a discharge'. The appeal can be made to a hospital manager (under Section 23) and/or to the Mental Health Review Tribunal (under Section 72).

ACTIVITY

1 Arrange to see an approved social worker who might be part of a care team in your agency or in your locality. Ask her which sections of the Mental Health Act she has applied in the course of her work during the past three months. Ask her to explain those sections to you.

2 Then ask her to tell you which compulsory detention that she was involved in she found most difficult, and why.

ACTIVITY

Ask several of your colleagues to join in a role play in which you imagine a client being taken into hospital or a police station against her or his will.

1 Try hard to imagine the experiences which you believe someone in those circumstances is going through. Then write down, independently of each other, all the feelings and thoughts which come to mind on having undergone the experience of being detained or given medical treatment against your will.

2 Now share what you have written. Discuss ways in which some of the distressing experiences during a process of sectioning could be minimised or avoided.

ACTIVITY

Find out which client (if any) in your care setting had to undergo enforced hospitalisation and compulsory medical treatment. Then ask if he or she will discuss the experience with you, but be ready to accept refusal.

Giving support to clients

One way of encouraging clients to talk about their experiences of distress is to begin by saying something like 'Would you like to talk about it?' Be patient and wait for a while for a response. If the client does not respond, do not just walk away or persist in questioning (by which the client might feel threatened); try to acknowledge his or her unwillingness to talk. For example, you could say: 'It must have been one of those experiences you'd rather not think about. It's all right if you'd rather not talk about it now.'

Being taken into a hospital and detained against one's will is undoubtedly a very distressing experience. One way of coping with such painful experiences and memories is to try and shut them out. Although this is not the best way of dealing with strong disturbing feelings, you should respect the clients' wishes and their needs, so be sensitive to their unwillingness to talk about them. Remember, you are a care worker and not a psychotherapist; if you attempt to bring to the surface deep painful feelings in your clients which you might not be able to deal with, you could make things worse. You will learn more about how to support the clients emotionally as you make progress in this book, on your course, and through your work with clients.

What else can you do to help?

You may have a client who has been hospitalised by compulsory detention, which means staying in a hospital, often for weeks or longer, unprepared. Your role as his worker might include visiting him in hospital and taking care of his practical affairs, such as bringing him clean clothes from his home or your care setting. Once the client leaves the hospital he will live in his community again, which could be your care setting. You should try to help him by making this transition as smooth as possible, for example by welcoming him and trying to make him feel at home if you work in a residential setting. But do not expect him to join in social activities as if nothing has happened, especially if the hospitalisation was long or particularly distressing.

TO THINK ABOUT

Imagine that you are experiencing mental distress similar to that described in the case study on page 29. If you had a choice that would include a wide range of professionals and treatments, relatives and friends, how and by whom would

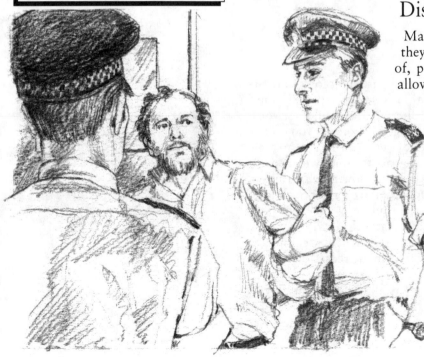

Distress at being handled by police

Many clients find it most distressing when they are taken to a hospital by, or in the presence of, police officers, which the Mental Health Act allows. They say that their symptoms get worse when they see a uniform. Being handled by a police officer suggests criminal behaviour and, as one client claimed, if you are innocent you will fight to protect yourself. Such a reaction is then interpreted as your being a danger to others. Compulsory medical treatment following such detention is then viewed by some clients as a punishment. In a recent radio discussion about the role of police in dealing with people experiencing mental distress, problems were expressed by both a police officer and a client. A constable acknowledged his inadequacy and lack of training to understand and deal with people experiencing mental distress. He felt this might lead to handling people inappropriately, perhaps by using too much force.

Some concerns about the Mental Health Act

Professionals and clients have expressed serious concerns about a number of issues surrounding this legislation. Some of these are:

- the way in which a person is treated during detention, as already described, especially the use of the police, which suggests criminality. This could be partly due to the lack of training of the police, but also because of the fear most people have – in rare cases justifiably – of someone acting in an unpredictable manner;
- the cultural differences in what constitutes 'normal' and 'disorderly' behaviour, as well as the narrow range of emotions and behaviours that individuals are permitted to express within our society;
- the cultural differences in expressing oneself; for example, a Black youth, brought to a psychiatric hospital after some trouble in a local pub, might reply to the question 'Do you know where you are?' with 'I am in Babylon.' A White British doctor might conclude that the answer is an indication the person has lost touch with reality, when in fact 'Babylon' is a popular metaphor among Afro-Caribbean youth for Western materialism and corruption;
- that people from other cultures are more likely to be detained because of racism (see Burke 1986). Those from Afro-Caribbean and Black backgrounds are over-represented in compulsory hospitalisation, and some agencies for these groups of clients employ lawyers for hospital discharge of clients;
- that compulsory medical treatment, especially by tranquillisers and ECT which can cause serious long-term damage, is limited, and that there should be other treatments at least equally accessible on the NHS;
- that some controversial forms of treatment, such as ECT, are used on the least powerful sections of society, such as older people and women.

Keeping your own feelings and views from your client

If you have strong views and feelings for or against a particular form of treatment and care, including the use of the Mental Health Act, try at all times not to influence your clients. This does not mean that you should not voice your views to those in power who can make changes, as long as you do not burden clients with your opinions which might be counterproductive to their immediate needs and experiences. Remember, they are the ones who need to get well, and they have the right to choose the kind of treatment which agrees with their individual or cultural beliefs. If they do not have a right to choose, such as during compulsory treatment, try to understand how they feel.

You must never tell a client not to take medication prescribed by the doctor. This does not mean that you should not support a client who complains that the medication is making her ill or is not working. In such cases, encourage her to talk to her doctor about the problem.

The best way you can help is to give the clients all the information you can about the services and treatments available to them. When a client decides on the kind of help she will accept, you should support her in that decision even if you do not approve of it for personal reasons.

An imperfect solution – better than none?

The Mental Health Act may well leave much to be desired. Yet as a society we do not currently know how best to take care of those who, because of severe symptoms of mental distress, cannot take care of themselves, or of those few who might be dangerous to others. Although they are very rare, acts of violence by clients do happen. Most of us would agree that, until we find other ways of coping with such problems, not having some kind of legislation in mental health would be both uncaring and irresponsible.

Further reading

★　A copy of *The Mental Health Act 1983* and the *Code of Practice* can be obtained by mail from PO Box 276, London SW8 5DT; by telephone 0171 873 9090; and by fax 0171 873 8200. They are also available from all HMSO bookshops.

For your information

★　Clients who have complaints about their care while in detention under the Mental Health Act 1983 (or their relatives) can contact the Mental Health Act Commission, Maid Marian House, 56 Houndsgate, Maid Marian Way, Nottingham NG1 6BG. Tel. 0115 950 4040.

2 Caring in the mental health setting

2.1 The care setting and care professionals

The new directives within community care strongly encourage that a multi-disciplinary, collaborative and multiagency approach be taken to ensure the best care for those who need it most. This will only be possible when the workers from the different agencies are clear about and have respect for their own and other professionals' roles. This is necessary in order to create good working conditions for successful team work and open communication free of bias and misunderstanding.

Where does mental health care take place?

People who use services for mental health difficulties can seek help in a number of different care settings. The range is constantly increasing, bringing a wider choice of treatment, including holistic and alternative approaches and self-help.

Traditionally, a psychiatric hospital or psychiatric wards within a general hospital have been major settings for mental health care. Other examples are:

- residential homes run by the voluntary or private sector, social services or health departments;
- supported lodgings (e.g. for the homeless) or sheltered housing;
- supported shared housing (e.g. run by housing associations);
- half-way homes (supported by staff), community homes and independent flats;
- day centres and day drop-ins (where clients can socialise and get informal staff support);
- a range of professional bodies and units offering counselling and psychotherapy;
- agencies offering rehabilitation through skills and work training for people with long-term mental distress;
- a range of helplines offering befriending and counselling, such as the Samaritans;
- counselling departments at colleges, universities and schools;
- centres for alternative treatment and holistic medicine;
- day and residential projects, including those for people of different ethnic origin;
- a range of self-support groups (e.g. for agoraphobia or schizophrenia; see section 1.2 and the list of support groups and organisations in Appendix 2).

ACTIVITY

1 Name at least three settings for mental health care.

2 Ask your colleagues to tell you about agencies they know where people who experience emotional difficulties can seek help.

3 Make enquiries about the existence of such agencies in your local area. Find out who runs those agencies (e.g. voluntary sector, private bodies, social services or health authorities).

ACTIVITY

1 Do you know the difference between the role of a psychiatrist and psychologist within mental health care? Complete the sentences below:

● A psychiatrist's training and job is . . .
● A psychologist's training and job is. . .

2 Find out about the role of a community psychiatric nurse (CPN).

Who are the carers?

The carers include a wide range of professionals, often with specialist training. For example, the core staff of psychiatric hospitals are medically trained professionals such as psychiatrists and psychiatric nurses. Social services departments, on the other hand, employ mainly social workers, social work assistants and welfare assistants – professionals who provide social care.

This does not mean that only one kind of professional is involved in each care setting. On the contrary, psychiatric hospitals also have social workers and social work assistants, and often psychologists, psychotherapists, occupational therapists, art therapists, voluntary befrienders and counsellors as well. Social services departments may also have other workers such as an art therapist or an occupational therapist.

Who does what?

A *psychiatrist* has a medical training. He or she is responsible for medical assessment and recommendations as well as for giving care, for example by prescribing medication or ECT (see section 1.2).

A *psychologist*, on the other hand, has a training in psychological methods of care. These are mainly to do with emotions and thinking. He or she gives psychological assessment, often by using tests, and administers psychological treatment such as cognitive–behaviour therapy or family therapy (see section 1.3).

A *community psychiatric nurse* cares for clients living in the community, but he or she can also run therapeutic programmes in a wide range of settings in the community.

Administering the law

Approved social workers (ASWs) are specially trained social workers who can be called to back up psychiatrists or GPs by signing the relevant forms for compulsory admission to hospital. In such circumstances they also support the clients and often take the role of the client's advocate.

Lawyers are sometimes involved in cases when a crime is committed by a person with mental distress, but also when there has been enforced admissions due to cultural misunderstanding, racism, sexual prejudice or other illegality.

Other carers

A warden in sheltered housing is often also a giver of support to vulnerable residents. Similarly, wardens or receptionists in women's refuge centres play a supportive role, as do workers in homes for single people (for example, housing associations) and youth workers.

ACTIVITY

Can you think of other people who give support to vulnerable people, yet whose main job is not to provide mental health care? Make a list to show who they are or where they might be employed.

Prevention versus long-term care and rehabilitation

All forms of help and support are valuable, whether they aim to prevent severe mental distress or relapse, or rehabilitate after hospitalisation and after long-term mental distress. It is important, however, to ensure that the right kind of help is given at the right time and in the most appropriate setting.

ACTIVITY

As you read through the following examples of clients receiving care, try to differentiate between clients receiving preventive care and those receiving rehabilitative care.

1 John has been hospitalised for ten years for severe depression and a series of attempts to end his life. He now attends a psychotherapy group at the outpatients' department of a psychiatric hospital.

2 Deborah is also a long-term sufferer who has been in and out of hospitals for her agoraphobia and depression; she has recently started to attend a self-help group.

3 Tim failed his finals at university and had an emotional crisis, described by his doctor as a breakdown. His moods, thinking and behaviour were erratic, and he could not concentrate or sleep. His doctor prescribed antidepressants, but Tim did not take them. He is now receiving support-counselling from a mental health social worker (who is a trained counsellor as well) at a day centre.

4 Michael has been living on the streets for a couple of years and is now staying in a hostel for homeless men. During the last visit by a doctor he was given medication to counteract his episodes of hallucinations, probably caused by his long-standing alcohol problem.

You probably guessed that Tim (example 3) is receiving preventive care which should prevent a decline in his mental health and consequent hospitalisation. The others are being helped on a continual long-term basis. But you could also say that psychotherapy for John (example 1) and the self-help group for Deborah (example 2) might lead to prevention of relapse and future hospitalisation.

The right kind of care for each client

If you and your care team cannot meet some or all of the needs of the client who turns to you, you should be able to help her by telling her about or referring her to other services outside your agency. It is also important that the client's preferences are sought, and that she takes an active part in decisions about her care whenever possible.

2.2 Receiving people for care

The way in which you receive clients into care will depend to a large extent on your care setting, its policies and guidelines, and your specific role within it. This section will discuss receiving clients through referrals, where your agency is also involved in the direct assessment of the clients' needs and has the power to make decisions about the provision of care.

Referral system

Receiving people into your care setting, either residentially or for a specific development or therapeutic programme and support, usually begins with a referral made by:

● a client's doctor or her psychiatrist;
● another professional, such as a warden of a hostel, a psychotherapist or a social worker from another agency;

- a family member or a partner;
- the client (self-referral).

Decisions about dealing with a referral are usually made collectively by the care team (all care workers of an agency). Most likely, such decisions will take place during one of the staff meetings.

Care team meetings

Every care setting has meetings to discuss clients and the roles which each worker is to carry out in relation to them. You may have attended some of the kinds of meetings described below.

Clients' referral meetings

Here, the clients most recently referred are discussed. If appropriate, the care workers are allocated tasks such as gathering more information, or arranging and conducting assessment interviews.

Clients' assessment meetings

These are held to continue the assessment of clients in the care of the agency, and to make evaluations and decisions about care plans.

Case conferences

These are meetings of the care workers from all agencies who contribute to caring for a particular client. They also include individuals such as the client's advocates (a friend, parent or voluntary befriender). All come together in order to share information and make a joint assessment which will form the basis for new decisions.

Staff/business meetings

Regular meetings of staff may be necessary to discuss the running of the care setting, covering matters such as buying supplies, health and safety needs, the duty rota, and clients' holidays and outings.

Ward rounds

In hospitals, the psychiatric consultant and relevant medical and non-medical workers will meet to discuss progress and make decisions (e.g. regarding discharge from the hospital) for clients who are hospitalised. The client may be invited for a chat to this meeting which is held on a hospital ward.

Other meetings

You will get to know about other meetings in your care setting and why they exist. These may include:

- key worker meetings with the client (see section 3.1);
- supervision meetings for care workers and their supervisors;
- clients' (users') meetings or patients' councils (see sections 3.8 and 5.4);
- staff training and staff support meetings.

ACTIVITY

1 Find out how many meetings you are expected to attend in the course of your work. State the frequency on a weekly or other basis.

2 Describe the nature of each kind of meeting.

3 Say why you think each kind is important.

4 Are you clear about your role during the various meetings?

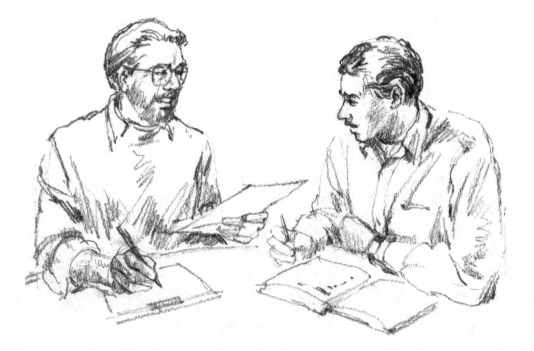

Supervision is an important part of mental health care

Keeping track of meetings

You should have a diary, which you use only for work, where you can keep track of your appointments, duties and tasks that you have undertaken. Whenever possible, estimate the time you need for each meeting and each task.

Towards successful meetings

For a meeting to be successful, communication between participants must be good. The effectiveness of communication during the meeting can improve greatly if you understand:

- the purpose of the meeting;
- your role;
- the role of others.

It is not easy to achieve the right balance between time spent on meetings and direct work with clients. You can best help if you remember the precious value of your time and that of all present. Remembering this, you should:

- take notes, letters, clients' files and other records that you might need with you;
- prepare to contribute to the meeting by thinking beforehand about what information you should share with those present and what you need to know from others;
- listen carefully to what is being said during every meeting;
- communicate clearly, verbally as well as in writing;
- remember to act promptly on tasks that you agreed to do during the meeting (such as make a phone call or write to the client).

ACTIVITY

1 Think of two circumstances when a meeting with other workers would be beneficial.

2 Could any of the existing meetings at your agency be done away with, made less frequent, shortened, or combined with another kind of meeting?

3 Make a list of other people who are not invited or not willing to attend meetings but whose contribution would be valuable.

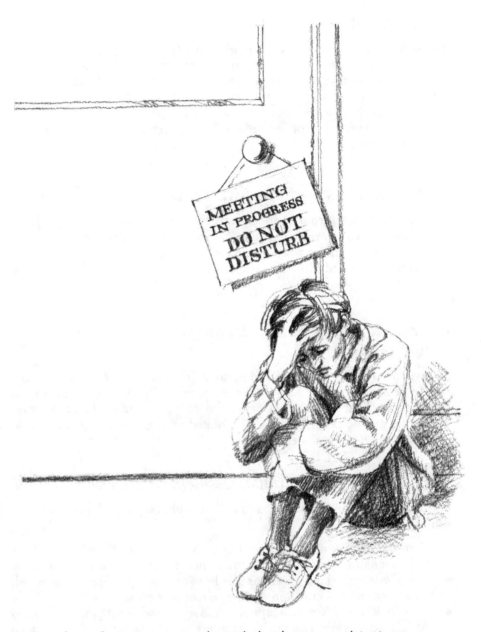

A client who needs support cannot understand what the carers are doing in so many meetings

2.3 Initial assessment interviewing

The process of caring usually goes through five stages. You can see a more detailed description of this process in section 3.9. Here are the main stages:

- assessment;
- planning;
- monitoring;
- reviewing;
- ending.

In this section we will concentrate on the first stage: assessment.

Assessment

Assessment of clients for care might not be within your role or that of your agency. If it is, a more senior professional will be responsible for it, although you might be asked to join him in this task. Even if you are not involved in assessment interviewing, the skills and knowledge required to conduct such an assessment will be of value to you in other situations, such as the assessment of individual development, therapeutic activities and programmes.

The initial assessment interview

Some agencies use forms where the structure of the interview is predetermined: the interviewer reads the questions to the client and fills in the answers. This may be appropriate when the objective is to gather factual information, such as name, date of birth and medical history, but in mental health care it is often not enough.

Information for a residential and a day care programme

You will need detailed medical and personal information for residential care, such as personal habits (e.g. does the client smoke?). It will be more important to assess the client's expectations for a day care programme, because if they are unrealistic the client will be disappointed or angry and mistrust you, so that future help might suffer.

Suggestions for an initial assessment interview

Information which you may need to collect could be put under a number of sub-headings:

- *Personal details*: name; date of birth; address; next of kin; name of the GP; name of the psychiatrist (consultant); name of the last care worker.
- *Social history*: where the client was born and brought up; ethnic origin; education; past occupation; family contacts; friends.
- *Mental health history*: hospital admissions and length of stay; dates of last admission; diagnosis; attempts at self-harm; treatment given (medical and psychological).
- *Physical health*: major operations and illness; hospitalisations; current medication; allergies; disability (if any); diet.

Before the interview

Before the interview, read all the information you have about the client, such as that given by other agencies. This will help you determine what else you might need to know.

If you are doing a joint assessment with another worker, meet before the interview to discuss what to ask, who will do the introduction and ask the questions, and who will record the information.

Do not forget to write to the client as soon as you set the date for the interview. You should include an information leaflet about the centre with a map of its location.

ACTIVITY

1 Write down the most important information you will need when admitting a new client into a residential care setting.

2 What information will be required for receiving clients into a specific programme (state which) of a day centre?

3 How are the two sets of information different? What are the reasons for the differences?

During the interview

Try and be as relaxed and informal as the circumstances permit. For example, make eye-contact with the client (which does not mean stare at her) rather than look down at your form or write all the time. You only need to write down personal details immediately. Try to remember the rest and write it down quickly as soon as the interview is over.

Points to remember

- Always prepare yourself for the interview.
- Book a quiet room and make sure that you are not interrupted.
- Be on time.
- Greet the client and introduce yourself. Explain the purpose of the interview, its duration, the procedure after the interview, and who will use the information.
- Tell the client about the confidentiality of information.
- Ask for permission if you need to write down notes.
- Always leave time for the client to ask questions or express concern.
- Ask the client for permission if you need to get in touch with her GP or a parent to either ask for or convey specific information.
- When you record information, make sure you record only the actual facts and not your interpretation of what the client says.

Inform the client about services available

Interviewing is never a one-way process. Remember that clients have a right to choose which services they prefer, but to do this they must know what services are available. Explain clearly what is offered within your care setting. In addition, it is always useful to have written information, such as leaflets, which new clients can take away and examine at their leisure.

After the interview

When you have recorded all the relevant information clearly and legibly, your next task is to share it with the care team and your supervisor. This could be done during the appropriate staff meeting. Make sure that your information is communicated clearly and accurately.

Once your care team has made a decision following the client's referral and assessment, the client should be informed without delay.

Assessment skills

Good assessment skills come with experience and learning. The specific skills needed will depend on the kinds of assessments used by your agency and on your role. But for all assessments you will need to learn how to:

- make clients feel at ease;
- communicate clearly;
- be a good listener;
- respect clients' need for privacy and confidentiality;
- know what questions to ask;
- record important information;

- remember important details;
- deal with clients' concerns and enquiries.

These are the skills which you need for all, or most, aspects of your work with clients. You probably have many of them already. This workbook and your practical experience will help you to sharpen those skills even more.

Assessment chart

What / who is assessed	By whom
1. Clients referred for social support (befriending/counselling or attending social/therapeutic activities at the centre)	Social worker(s); a counsellor; a member of a care team
2. Clients' suitability for a developmental group activity	Group leader(s)
3. Progress of a specific care programme (review)	Key worker, alone or with professionals responsible for clients' rehabilitation
4. Clients' eligibility for the forthcoming centre holiday	Team decision on eligibility criteria; named workers to assess individual clients
5. Suitability of clients who apply to help out in the centre (voluntary or paid work)	Named worker who co-ordinates the work applied for, supported by the team and/or his supervisor

ACTIVITY

1 Draw a chart to show: (a) what kinds of assessments are carried out by your agency, and (b) who is responsible for each of them. (See the example below.)

2 Take two examples of assessments from your chart and draw another chart listing which tasks are needed for each assessment. Ask colleagues to help you if you are not sure.

2.4 Gathering, storing and sharing information

Gathering, storing and sharing information about services and clients is an integral part of your work. How you do this can have a significant effect on the clients' welfare and well-being and on the running of your agency.

Information kept in your workplace

Your care setting might keep information about:

- *the clients*: biographical details and personal history, medical records including test results, and details of the care or services which they receive;
- *the care setting*: its policies, statutory obligations and practices; its budget including the cost of services it offers; information regarding other professionals, stock records and so on;
- *its employees*: personal details such as name, home address, confidential medical reports and work assessment reports.

Right to privacy: security of information

All individuals have a right to privacy and dignity. Keeping information secure, such as the files held on clients, is one way of preserving this basic human right and need. This means you should keep the filing cabinets locked whenever they are not in use and when other unauthorised staff, visitors or clients

ACTIVITY

1 How secure is the information kept on clients in your care setting? Discuss this issue with colleagues.

2 Describe your current practice for keeping information confidential. Then suggest how it can be improved.

could walk in. You should also mark all confidential reports and other personal details 'Confidential', so that they never get mixed up with other kinds of information, or get misplaced and lost.

Confidentiality of information

It is essential that you understand what confidentiality of information about clients means and how it is practised in your care setting. Whether you receive information from a third party such as another agency (written, oral or electronic), or from the client directly, personal and health details should be stored safely and not shown to anyone who is not supposed to be informed. Never give details about your clients to anyone outside your care network, such as your friends or family members.

If you are approached by an unidentified person from another agency, always check the person's identity. Make sure you know why the confidential information is required. When you suspect the caller's motives and cannot establish his identity, refuse politely, explaining the agency's policy on confidentiality.

Data Protection Act 1984

Check with your supervisor to ensure that you follow the procedures and guidelines set out by your employer and by legislation known as the Data Protection Act 1984. According to this Act, all agencies who use computerised systems for keeping clients' records are required to register with the Data Protection Agency to prevent the potential abuse of confidential information by unauthorised persons.

Open access to information

Your agency may have an open access policy whereby clients have a right to see their confidential files under the Access to Personal Files Act (introduced in 1987). The Act does not include information on files from before 1989, although this is presently under revision. On viewing their files, clients have a right to correct any errors and to add their statement on any disputed issues.

Open access does not mean that you can show the clients their files at any time; there is a procedure for this, and your senior colleagues and supervisor will advise you more closely if any of your clients have expressed a wish to see their files. A client might need some counselling prior to reading her file.

Recording personal information

Bearing in mind that clients might read what you write about them, always remember to take particular care how you record such information. Ask yourself:

- Am I complying with the guidelines of my work setting and its policies regarding what and how I should record information?
- Am I stating the facts (when reporting the client's behaviour, for example) or am I confusing the facts with my interpretation?
- Am I using the right language and tone to show sensitivity to the client who might be reading this?

The final test is to read what you have written and imagine that you are reading another worker's description of yourself. Do you find something there offensive, inaccurate or insufficiently explained? Could your behaviour or what you said be misunderstood when taken out of the context in which it appeared?

Gathering, recording and sharing information

Whenever information regarding clients, other professionals or agencies is gathered or shared, you should always be careful to ascertain:

- the purpose of seeking or sharing such information;
- the clarity/legibility of its recording and its transmission;
- the importance of the information and the timing of any necessary action: for example, whether you should disturb a meeting or your supervisor to pass on a message, or when to contact the client's doctor;
- statutory and agency requirements: for example, a prompt and accurate recording of accidents and incidents in accordance with the agency's policy and legal requirements, such as the Health and Safety at Work Act 1974.

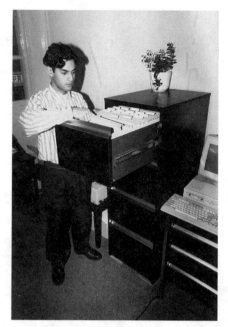

Everything in its place

You should also watch the manner in which you give or receive information. For example, you must ensure confidentiality and security at all times, including during transmission. Make sure that the language used is clear and appropriate for the individual receiving the information. Adopt an anti-discriminatory attitude in dealing with information – be sensitive to an individual's cultural beliefs, observing the principles of equal opportunity and all clients' rights to service, dignity and respect.

ACTIVITY

Ask a colleague to help you in this role-playing exercise.

After becoming familiar with the policy and guidelines of your agency on this issue, let your colleague take the role of a difficult and to you unknown caller who rings up demanding confidential information regarding one of your clients. Go through the procedure of speaking to him or her, and if necessary repeat the role play until you are confident that you can refuse the immediate request in a manner both helpful to the caller and in accordance with the practice and policy of your care setting.

2.5 Using communication and observation skills

Communication is more than the exchange of words from one person to another. We communicate in many ways: the way we dress, our gestures and postures, and the tone and volume of our voice when we speak. We also communicate by the way in which we choose or are compelled to live: the kind of house or neighbourhood we live in, the people we have for friends, the job we do, the kind of car we drive. Everything we do seems to communicate something about ourselves.

Verbal communication

During your work you will use words both in speaking and writing. To be skilful in verbal communication you need to:

- speak clearly and fluently;
- speak at the volume appropriate for the context: for example, use a quiet voice when the client is distressed, and a louder voice when you are in a large room or in the open with a group of clients and need to ensure that everyone hears you;
- choose words which are appropriate for the person to whom they are spoken: for example, do not use professional jargon with clients;
- keep to the point without jumping from one subject to another;
- use pauses appropriately so that the other person knows when you have stopped to think and wish to continue or when you have finished speaking;
- be aware of any sexist or racist language which you might have adopted as a matter of habit.

Non-verbal communication

This includes all but the actual words used during communication. It can be further divided into three parts: paraverbal cues (for example, the tone or quality of the voice), body 'language' (posture and body movements), and facial expression.

Paraverbal cues

Our voice can be loud, quiet or somewhere between these two extremes. The speed with which we speak can vary, as can the pitch of our voice and the stress we place on certain words. Your voice can take on different tones such as joking, angry, playful, sad, serious, sympathetic or threatening. All these qualities form paraverbal cues which act as signs. They can disclose the way you really feel about something or someone and reveal your emotional state.

CASE STUDY

A client in your care setting has visited her parents over the weekend, and on her return you ask how her visit went. 'Fine', she replies in a dull voice. You pursue this and ask if she had a good time.

After a pause (which suggests uncertainty) she answers 'Yes, I had a good time'. Her voice is slow and quiet, and she uses a downward inflection which can suggest disappointment. You notice the discrepancy between the words used and how the client expresses herself. Do you believe she really had a good time? Or does your 'sixth sense' tell you she is only being polite and not telling you the true course of the weekend visit?

Some guidelines

By becoming more aware of the volume, rapidity of speech and tone of your voice during your interaction with clients, you can begin to modify them and so improve communication.

- A calm voice can have the effect of soothing and absorbing a client's anxieties. It can counteract agitation or aggression.
- By not rushing to fill in momentary pauses when a client stops talking (especially an incomplete sentence), you communicate patience and suggest that you care.

- Understanding that people from different ethnic and cultural backgrounds may use a different volume or tone of voice can prevent you from labelling them as aggressive if their voice is louder than you are used to, or unco-operative if their voice is slow and quiet.

Body language

Think again about the client in the previous case study, whose tone of voice suggests the opposite meaning from the words she uses. Perhaps you did not look at her as she spoke. If you did, you would have seen her hand covering her mouth as she finished speaking. A hand over the mouth in Western cultures usually indicates that a person is hiding something; perhaps the client is thinking something which she would rather be silent about. Body language includes:

- body posture and gestures;
- physical distance or proximity;
- eye-contact and facial expression.

Like paraverbal cues, body posture can show your real attitude to the client or a colleague even if your words say something different.

Some guidelines
For good communication you should:

- stand or sit facing the person to whom you are talking, at a distance appropriate for the nature of the relationship and the client's culture (see section 2.6) – further apart with clients and colleagues, closer with family members and partners;
- try to be at eye level – sitting on a higher chair may suggest your power over the client;
- lean the upper half of your body slightly forward – this shows interest in the speaker;

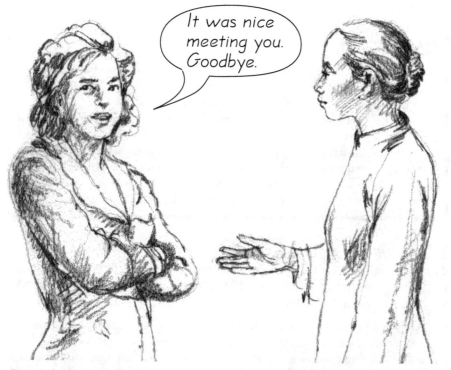

Do you believe the sincerity of the person on the left? Make sure that your words confirm your non-verbal cues

- make eye-contact but do not stare – in Western cultures the speaker makes less eye-contact than the listener;
- keep your limbs, especially arms, uncrossed – this indicates 'openness', that is, willingness to listen and to communicate;
- avoid using too many hand movements when speaking – they can distract the listener;
- avoid playing with your hair, a pen or other object because this communicates boredom or nervousness;
- avoid looking at your watch – such a gesture gives the impression that you are impatient or bored.

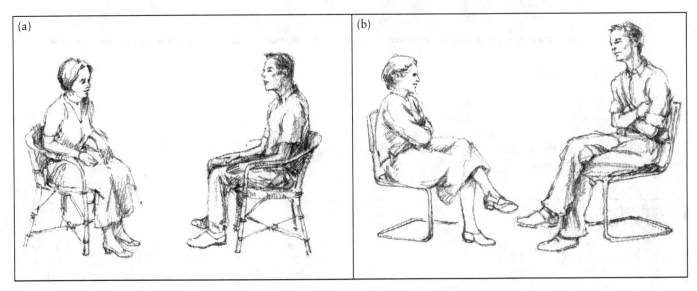

(a) 'Open' and (b) 'closed' body postures: the first encourages while the second discourages communication

Facial expression

The face is the focal point during personal encounters, so you need to consider how to use it most effectively. For example, some people smile even when they speak about something sad, or they laugh when their words indicate anger. They may hide their true negative feelings because they have learned, as children, that those around them will like them only if they smile and express happiness.

A need for approval and fear of rejection can later produce a fixed facial expression, often without the person being aware of it. As a carer you must realise how an inappropriate facial expression, for example when a client communicates and feels the opposite of what your face reflects, can cause adverse reactions. Even if the client does not react overtly, your rapport, and so your chances of establishing a good working relationship with him, will suffer.

Some guidelines

Your facial expression should reflect that of your client, with the intensity appropriate for the subject you are discussing. There are exceptions, as for example when the other person does not show appropriate emotions; in such cases your more suitable facial expression can help the client to get in touch with and reveal his or her true feelings.

If a client expresses sadness, your mirroring this in your facial expression will convey sympathy. If the client communicates happiness, seeing this reflected in your face will intensify it.

ACTIVITY

1 Ask a colleague or friend to take part in a role play in which he or she tells you about an event (e.g. a news item or a fictional event) of an unfortunate, sad nature. Listen first and then look in the mirror to note your facial expression. (If the mirror makes you too self-conscious, ask a third colleague to act as an observer.) Is your face reflecting the feelings which the event arouses?

2 Now change roles so that you give an account of an upsetting event from the news. Watch yourself in the mirror while you do it. You can adjust to a more appropriate facial expression if you feel a need for it. Your colleague can do the same exercise after you.

3 Ask your colleague to describe the emotions that your face shows while you close your eyes and think vividly about an event or personal experience. Do this exercise for several kinds of emotions (fear, grief, happiness) and then swap roles.

Observation skills

Observation is more than having your eyes open. You must be consciously aware of what you see, which cannot happen if your mind is somewhere else. Observation skills consist of the use of all senses: seeing, hearing, smelling, touching and tasting. The extent to which you use each of these will depend on what you need to know.

ACTIVITY

Read the following case study, then answer the questions set below.

Case study

Geoff Myrth moves into his flat from residential mental health care accommodation. Five months later you receive a call from his relative, who expresses concern that Geoff may not be coping with the everyday tasks of independent living. You pay Geoff a visit, intending to carry out a reassessment interview, which you need to produce a report for your agency. Geoff shows you inside the flat and you take a seat he offers you in the hall. You proceed to look at the necessary forms, anxious that you should not forget anything. You read out questions such as: 'Did you pay your last heating bill?', 'Do you shop and cook regularly?', 'When did you last clean your flat and do your laundry?', and fill in the appropriate boxes. According to the client's answers everything seems fine and, barely glancing around, you leave the premises satisfied that you completed the interview fully.

1 What did you forget during this interview?

2 How would you go about making sure that your visit fulfils the purpose of reassessing the client's ability to cope with the tasks of everyday living?

You might think that this case study gave an exaggerated description of events in which the care worker (could this ever be you?) forgets to make observations concerning the client's home environment. In this example, observation would be the best way of finding out how someone is coping with various tasks of independent living. This is not just because clients' self-reports are not to be trusted. Clients who give all positive answers, despite evidence of the contrary, may genuinely believe that they are coping; their personal standards and understanding of what is regarded as coping well may be very different from the accepted cultural norms. Or they may have a good reason to hide the facts from you, such as the fear of a return to institutionalisation and a loss of independence.

Sometimes you will have to be creative, diplomatic and tactful in order to make your observations as unobtrusive or as kind as possible, showing respect for the client's privacy, yet doing your job as well as you can.

Why make observations?

Some reasons for observation are:

- ensuring the safety and security of clients, yourself and other people, including that of visitors and the general public;
- assessing the clients' needs and monitoring their development;
- making informal re-evaluation of your work with clients;
- monitoring the clients' changes in moods and behaviour so that, if the mental health symptoms become worse, you can alert others to take necessary measures to help the client.

When to use observation skills

Use observation skills to gain an overview of any situation you are in with your clients, monitoring their rehabilitation while also ensuring everybody's safety. For example, you should observe:

- what individual clients can and cannot do for themselves, especially if they have been institutionalised for a time;
- clients' interaction with each other, and their reactions to other people and to what others say or do. Noticing inappropriate behaviour promptly (for instance, when one client becomes aggressive towards another) will enable you to intervene, ensuring safety, security and a harmonious social environment;
- clients' reactions to you during your personal meetings (known as one-to-one interactions). This will help you establish a good rapport – the basis of a good working relationship;
- what is generally going on in your work setting. Any irregularities or unsound practice by a colleague, visitor or anyone else should be reported to the appropriate person in charge.

Observation is not interpretation

Communicating your observations and your concerns based upon them to other professionals is an integral part of making the most of your observation skills. But be sure that, in communicating your observations (which includes writing them down), you give an account of the facts and not your interpretation of what you saw.

How we see and recall things

It is not uncommon for the same events to be described differently by different observers. Our background, education, past experience and beliefs, as well as emotional states, can all influence what or how we see – or rather what we register and recall. For example, a parent who believes that her child is good and well behaved may reject any evidence to the contrary provided by teachers. To avoid making similar mistakes, become aware of your personal value system and your stereotypes which might influence the way you see individual clients (see also sections 2.6 and 2.7).

Be aware how you communicate

Observation, listening (see section 3.3) and communicating go hand in hand. All three are essential elements of good communication. To achieve this you should learn to be aware of the verbal and non-verbal aspects of your own as well as your clients' communication.

Some people with mental health problems are very aware of non-verbal aspects of communication, so they can sense when others are not genuine. Their trust in such people will be diminished, which can have serious consequences on their care.

Everyone can benefit from learning more about how to be a good communicator. If you do this, you will see the reward of such effort both in work and in daily life.

2.6 Communicating: individual differences and race

Every man is like all other men in certain respects, like some other men, and like no other men.

Kluckhohn and Stodtbeck, 1961

Although it is true that as human beings there is more that binds us than separates us, we should not ignore the uniqueness of each individual. You should always strive to understand your clients and accept that which makes them different. This may, at times, not be easy, especially when accepting some people might challenge your religious and cultural background, your beliefs and your misconceptions. This section and the next will help you to gain knowledge and awareness of two poorly understood differences among people – multiracial issues and homosexuality – which in conjunction with mental health distress can represent quite a challenge for the client as well as for the carer.

> **ACTIVITY**
>
> *1* Make a list of ways in which people are different.
>
> *2* Do such differences influence the mental health care of clients and, if so, how?

People like us

Most of us feel more comfortable when we are with people who are similar to us; the greater the similarity, the more at ease we feel. This is because we feel safer with the familiar; we know what to expect and what is expected from us. Besides, by knowing more people like ourselves, people with the same cultural and racial backgrounds, religion, dress, age, sexual orientation and lifestyle, we are having our own identities confirmed and reinforced. Support of this kind is good for maintaining our identity and self-esteem.

How differences affect clients

In section 1.1 we discussed the problems of social stigma and stereotyping which people with mental health difficulties experience. As well as these problems imposed by society at large, clients are faced with additional problems if they happen to belong to one of the minority groups defined by race, sexual orientation or lifestyle.

The psychological effect of being rejected for what one is, or being perceived as inferior, is that eventually the person begins to believe he is truly inferior. The person may then reject an important part of his identity, such as being Black or being gay, and feel further alienated, which is contrary to the aim of mental health care and contrary to being a whole human being.

The real problem

You must be cautious here; it is not differences as such that are the real problem, but how society and the people around the individual accept or reject them. Unfortunately, many people are not yet sufficiently educated to view differences as positive, enriching the whole of humanity.

Get to know about clients' differences

Section 1.1 warned against stereotyping, but it is not easy to know when you are communicating prejudice, lack of accurate knowledge and misunderstanding of any group of people of whom you have limited experience and knowledge. This is why you should strive to learn about people who do not belong to the same group as you do, especially people whose particular experience is different from the majority.

Acknowledge existence of prejudice

If we wish to understand and develop the skills necessary to deal with multicultural and multiracial issues, we need first to acknowledge that people of the majority culture (White British) have an advantage in most aspects of living. They have power, resources and socio-economic prestige.

The fact that in a democratic society there are laws to deal with those who practise racial discrimination, and also discrimination based on disability or sexual orientation, does not mean that people's attitudes, especially unconscious and deeply imbedded ones, have changed. This means that discrimination and prejudice still go on, often in subtle ways that are not noticed or acknowledged.

Mental health care is for all

Whether or not you belong to the dominant culture, your duty as a care worker is to show that you are willing to care for all clients, irrespective of racial, economic, religious or other differences. You will only be able to do this satisfactorily if you learn how to care for people whose cultural beliefs, traditions, religion and expectations are different from your own. This could be, for example, an Asian, Irish or Black client living in a predominantly English or White British community.

ACTIVITY

Select a client from your care setting whose cultural, racial or religious background is different from your own.

1 Note down your (confidential) thoughts and feelings regarding this client. Be as specific as you can.

2 Note down what you know about the group (e.g. race) to which that client belongs. Try hard to distinguish the facts about it as opposed to hearsay, stereotyping or the images portrayed through the media.

3 Now make a list of things you would like to learn about the client's background, bearing in mind his mental health needs. Consider how you can set about acquiring such knowledge.

4 Be sure to destroy everything you have written for 1 and 2 so that it cannot be read by the client or others.

How to learn about someone's culture

The best way of learning about someone's culture is directly from people themselves. Having a friend or colleague from the culture to which your client belongs means you can learn in an informal and interesting way about customs, social etiquette, family relationships, verbal and non-verbal ways of communicating, and so on. You can also learn from literature, newspapers and magazines, or by participating in local events such as religious festivals. For example, most forms of worship and the socialising that follows are free to all; a visit to a Sikh temple on Sunday may include your being invited to share the common lunch.

Some cultural differences

Verbal communication

If a client does not speak sufficient English, you should seek an interpreter with the same regional dialect. Lack of resources often means that children or relatives of a client are employed to translate. This practice is not adequate in mental health care because of the confidentiality of some sensitive information.

Non-verbal communication: eye-contact

Some Asian people do not engage in much eye-contact. Instead, looking down or away from the speaker is a way of showing respect. In some Black cultures looking at the speaker during conversation is not necessary, because being in the same room is sufficient.

Attempts to make eye-contact might be seen as aggressive to some Black people. Note that this is usually the opposite in White European cultures, where not making eye-contact could be misinterpreted as being impolite or aggressive. Latin Americans and Arabs, however, tend to engage in mutual gaze more than Europeans.

Physical distance and contact

In some Black cultures, it is common to engage in spontaneous touching when in conversation. Touching, including hugging and holding hands with those of the same sex, is also accepted by most Arabs and by some people of the Balkans.

ACTIVITY

Since people from non-White groups experience being in the minority every day by living in a British White society, this activity is for British White care workers only.

Find a geographical area accessible to where you live or work which is densely populated with people from one of the major ethnic groups in the UK, such as Black African, Afro-Caribbean or Asian cultures. Choose an activity within the area, such as shopping in shops owned or staffed by these ethnic groups. Or if you have a friend there, you might be able to get yourself invited to a party or religious festival. If possible, make sure that you are the only person from the White British culture present. Once there, concentrate hard to be aware of and to remember your feelings and how you are treated.

Tell your experiences to a colleague, describing how you felt, other people's reactions to your presence, your level of comfort, and the spontaneity of your and others' behaviour.

Self-disclosure

Telling another person (who could be a stranger) about yourself is not an accepted thing to do in some cultures. You may need to explain why you need such information, and share something about yourself first, to build trust and credibility.

Do not overemphasise the cultural or racial differences

Sometimes, rather than ignoring an individual's ethnic or racial differences, people give far too much emphasis to them. Take care not to do this, because it can alienate the person completely. Neither is it wise to treat such people as helpless victims of prejudice because they are different, although some individuals might feel that way. This is not helpful; people need others to believe in them and in their ability to stand up for themselves, sometimes with the help of those who understand and genuinely accept their differences.

For your information

★ Your local library contains a section with books on different countries. The section on anthropology has literature on the customs and ways of life for different cultures and races. The library should also hold magazines, newspapers (e.g. *The Voice*) and journals used by the communities living in your area. These can also be bought from your local newsagent.

★ The *Ethnic Switchboard* can locate language interpreters and offers translating services, while the *Ethnic Study Group* gives monthly seminars and offers training, support and supervision to mental health workers in the London area. Further details can be obtained from: Ethnic Study Group and Ethnic Switchboard, Co-ordinating Centre for Community and Health Care, 28 Lessingham Avenue, London SW17 8LU. Tel. 0181 682 0216.

2.7 Communicating: sexual orientation

The issue of clients' relationships is likely to come up in your work. This might be about their past, as in broken relationships and divorce. You may also have to help clients by supporting them during their current relationships. For the majority, an intimate relationship signifies romantic and sexual ties with those of the opposite sex. Yet about one in ten men in the general population is gay, while the figures are slightly lower for women. This fact makes it natural to expect a proportional representation of homosexuality within a mental health care setting, among both clients and care workers. However, it is reasonable to assume that many heterosexual care workers – just like the general population – have little understanding and experience in relating to people who are homosexual.

Until recently homosexuality was totally taboo. The social stigma which still surrounds this issue is slowly losing its power, but this is not to say that it no longer exists. The result has been that many people with homosexual feelings have remained silent, for fear that they would be rejected, bullied, discriminated against, and perhaps even physically abused.

This section aims to dispel some myths and stereotypes, and to enable you to have a better understanding so that you can learn to relate to homosexual clients, accept and value them as human beings, and feel comfortable while caring for them.

Language

Homosexual is a term used to describe people whose affection and sexual attraction are for those of the same sex as themselves.

Research shows (see Appendix 3) that this term tends to make people think of men, although it also includes women. Most people feel it is a clinical term. The majority of men defined as homosexuals prefer the term *gay*; women prefer to be called *lesbians*, although some wish to be referred to as 'gay women'.

Bisexual men and women can be attracted to both genders to a similar degree.

When is a person gay?

Sometimes it is an individual who defines himself or herself as gay. Gay people are not necessarily exclusively attracted to those of the same sex. Many have had or are having relationships with both sexes, but are distinctly more attracted to those of the same gender as themselves. Someone can be gay even if he or she is in a heterosexual relationship without having had a sexual experience with a same sex partner, but instead fantasises about it regularly, especially during sexual intercourse. Recent research, published in *The Psychologist* (1995), estimates that about 50 per cent of gay men and women in Britain are married.

Some gay men and lesbians choose to marry because:

- they want children;
- they need social approval rather then rejection;
- they hope that their attraction for the same sex partner might go away – which it does not.

> **TO THINK ABOUT**
>
> What do you think are the reasons for such a high proportion (50 per cent) of gay people being married?

Homophobia

Homophobia is an intense fear of being in contact with gay men and lesbians. This fear is often the cause of the hostility which some heterosexual people express towards people with a homosexual orientation.

Preference or orientation?

Homosexuality is not a matter of preference, but of discovery that you are attracted to those of your own gender. The only choice you may have is whether or not to act in accordance with what you feel.

To 'come out' or not?

The expression 'to come out' is used to describe the process when gay men and lesbians no longer hide their attraction to those of the same gender, but openly announce that they are gay or lesbian.

This is a big step to take, not least because the reaction of people close to them is often that of shock, rejection, and even parental disowning. The legal (as in marriage), social and religious support which heterosexuals have does not apply to them. Yet, despite the risk of being rejected by those closest to them, the evidence exists that those who 'come out' tend to be better adjusted both socially and psychologically. They no longer need to sacrifice or suppress their natural feelings, and they free themselves from the stress and fear of being found out.

ACTIVITY

Read the following case study and then jot down:

- your reactions to the client's revelation about her sexuality;
- what sort of help and advice, if any, you would be tempted to give her.

Case study

Miriam is 29 and has been working for a small trading company for nine years. She has told no one about her attraction for her own gender, and over the years she has made up various excuses about why she is not in a relationship (her office colleagues and friends expect this to be with a man) and why she never brings a man to functions and parties. Finally, her colleagues and friends began to make jokes about her celibacy, and they tried using devious means to match Miriam with various men. Naturally she always rejected them, and her friends became quite challenging towards her, making her feel that 'there was something wrong with her'.

The greatest pressure came from her mother, who was terminally ill. She pleaded with Miriam, her only child, to hurry up and start a family – to 'make mother happy before she dies'. Miriam could not bear this pressure and, in distress, sought support at the local day centre.

No longer able to keep her secret locked inside her, she tells you about her lesbian inclinations. She also wants you to tell her how she should proceed; should she tell her mother the truth, or remain feeling guilty the rest of her life if her mother dies in ignorance? Should she tell colleagues and friends – surely they would reject her or make fun of her? Yet, she could no longer go back to work and face their continual pressure.

Support your clients: do not decide for them

You should never give advice or put pressure on your gay clients to 'come out', because they are the best judges as to whether or not they could cope with all the possible consequences. Instead, support them by standing by them whichever decision they make. You may well be the first, or one of the first people whose acceptance and non-judgement they need. They may treat you as a test of whether or not the world outside will understand and accept them.

- Never tell clients that their gay impulses will go away.
- Never say that it is wrong to have such feelings.
- Never suggest that they should try to meet people of the opposite sex.
- Never suggest that their parents will accept them if they 'come out' – you cannot know this for sure.

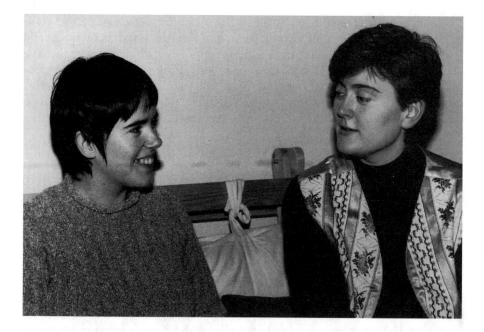

- Never doubt their revelation about their sexuality by probing in a way which may suggest that they have not tried hard enough to form a relationship with the opposite sex.
- Never make assumptions that being gay means having AIDS.

Some myths and stereotypes

Below are some of the most commonly held erroneous views and unhelpful generalisations about gay people.

- Gay men and lesbians take roles similar to 'husbands' and 'wives'. (This is not true; their relationships are more flexible and roles are negotiable.)
- Gay men are on the whole 'effeminate', while lesbians are 'butch'.
- Gay people want to be of the opposite gender.
- Gay people hate those of the opposite sex. (In fact, they often make good friends with them, as there is no sexual tension between them to interfere with the feeling of true friendship.)
- All that a gay man needs is hormone injections or to meet 'the right woman'.
- All that a lesbian needs is to meet a 'real man'.

How you can help

Showing acceptance, understanding and warmth are the best ways to communicate your acknowledgement that everyone has a right to express his or her identity through relationships which feel natural to them. An open body posture (see section 2.5) will help to communicate your willingness to understand and a genuine interest in your clients.

However, if you find homosexuality too difficult to understand, and so feel uneasy with gay clients, do not hesitate to talk to your supervisor confidentially – even if he or she happens to be gay. Your gay supervisor should be more resourceful in dealing with homophobia than your gay clients.

> **ACTIVITY**
>
> Ask your colleagues to take part in a discussion which aims to find ways of helping clients in your care setting overcome homophobia.
>
> For example, you could arrange to have a discussion about gay and lesbian issues, especially in relation to a mental health care setting, during which clients could express their concerns and ask questions. This might include a role-play exercise which would help the clients learn to empathise with people whose lifestyle and sexuality they do not understand. Or you might wish to invite a speaker from another organisation to give a talk.

Should you find the issue too difficult, a gay client could be allocated to another worker, giving you more time to gain further understanding. It is far better to be honest and acknowledge your limitations than to pretend otherwise. Remember, clients have a way of knowing when a worker is not genuine, which can have a damaging effect on their rehabilitation.

For your information

★ The *Gay and Lesbian Switchboard* is a network of telephone lines spread throughout the country offering free counselling to gay men and women. Information and help (24 hour) is available on 0171 837 7324. Your library or local telephone directory will have details of your local helpline.

2.8 Promoting equality in care

ACTIVITY

1 Read the list below which describes a number of clients from different backgrounds. Three of them will be your responsibility for overall care. Which three would you choose?

- a divorced, middle-class English woman
- a male ex-offender (convicted for hard drugs)
- an HIV positive father of three small children
- a Rastafarian youth
- a member of the National Front
- an older Asian woman with poor English-speaking ability
- a strict Moslem man who insists on daily prayers
- a lesbian
- a physically disabled, working-class man

2 Are you aware of your reasons for choosing these particular clients? If so, list them.

3 Which three clients from the same list would you least like to care for, and why?

Promoting equality in care means that you must follow legislation and charters concerning individual rights. Your organisation and its employees are responsible for ensuring non-discriminatory practice under the following:

- the Race Relations Act;
- equal opportunities policies;
- the Sex Discrimination Act;
- the Rehabilitation of Offenders Act;
- the Disabled Persons Act;
- the Fair Employment (Northern Ireland) Act;
- the Patient's Charter.

According to the Race Relations Act 1976, you or your colleagues would be breaking the law if you discriminated against someone on racial grounds. Similarly, the Disabled Persons Act 1986 ensures that you and your agency provide a range of services to disabled people and their carers. These and other Acts mentioned in this workbook, such as the Health and Safety at Work Act, apply to a mental health setting as they do in all other caring contexts. The Mental Health Act and the NHS and Community Care Act (see Chapter 1) should also be applied in a non-discriminatory manner. This means that you should apply your care, as outlined by the law and policies of your agency, to all people irrespective of their:

- race;
- religion;
- political belief;
- culture;
- age;
- HIV status;
- physical health status;
- mental health status;
- physical ability;
- sexuality;
- criminal record.

Your role within the care setting will determine your level of responsibilities in this area.

Your preferences regarding clients

Your preference for clients from certain backgrounds is natural; you might feel that being more familiar with the client's culture, race, class, lifestyle and religion would help. You might think that you would find it difficult to have a good working relationship with a client whose origins, personal history and culture are alien to you.

Alternatively, you might dislike and avoid people who, for example, belong to a religion which you do not approve of or who have been law-breakers. Like many people, you might even wish to punish people from backgrounds of which you do not approve.

Caring is non-judgemental

Being a caring professional has nothing to do with passing judgement on people or punishing them for what you, using your own set of values and beliefs, might view as 'bad' behaviour. By not being willing to offer the same standard of care to all clients irrespective of who they are or what they may have been guilty of, you are in fact punishing them. And that, clearly, is not your job. As a care worker you are asked to put aside all prejudices you may harbour and, instead, to look at clients as individuals with specific care needs.

Overt discrimination

Overt discrimination refers to behaviours or actions which are easily observed.

Example
Your agency has money to take only 12 clients on a holiday, and so certain criteria have to be applied for selection. One criterion is that a client has to have no other means of going on holiday – no family member to take him or her and no finance. According to this criterion, a Nigerian client in your care would be suitable for selection. However, you and your colleagues agree that you do not wish to spend public money on 'people from abroad'. Instead you give the place to a White British client who has already been on a holiday that year, paid for by his wealthy parents. You apologise to the Nigerian man, saying that all the places have been filled. Your overt behaviour in rejecting the Nigerian client shows discrimination on racial grounds.

Covert discrimination

Overt discrimination is easy to notice, so most people avoid it for fear of having to pay the price of breaking the law. Covert discrimination is therefore more common. By being subtle, people can still discriminate but can do it more frequently. They also feel safer this way because it is more difficult to be accused of discriminatory practice. This explains how laws against discrimination have not stopped people being prejudiced against some individuals, whether on racial, disability, sexuality or other grounds.

Example
Imagine that you have correctly selected the Nigerian client for the holiday paid for by your agency. However, you resent the fact that you have to follow anti-discriminatory policies and take this out on the client. During the holiday you ignore him whenever he approaches you, or your response to him is

minimal. Your body language and other non-verbal forms of communication are those of rejection and disapproval. You also make sure he gets the worst seat in the dining room for meals and the smallest food portions. All this is done in a way which makes it difficult for an outsider to notice your discrimination.

Discriminating is uncaring

Discriminatory behaviour, however subtle or covert, has a negative impact on your clients. They feel rejected and their self-esteem suffers. Although most other people will not notice the covert expression of your prejudices, those against whom it is directed will. This is because they have experienced such rejections often, and so learned how to recognise its various disguises as a way of survival in an environment where prejudice is rife and becoming more sophisticated all the time.

Awareness is the first step to equality

Much of our routine behaviour is automatic, driven by habit and deep-seated attitudes, beliefs and values. In the previous example you would have probably denied your discriminatory treatment of the Nigerian client were you confronted. Your denial might have been sincere, because you lacked awareness of your attitudes and behaviour.

Self-examination as a skill in caring

The first step to applying the principle of equality when giving care is being brave enough to look at your values. You must be able, honestly, to examine your attitudes, thoughts and feelings, and your beliefs concerning individual clients, their families and the community from which they come.

After all, most of our attitudes come from 'outside' – passed on to us through our upbringing. A child has no choice in what to believe and what to reject as a false representation of reality, as she learns from what is given to her. Besides, the picture of 'reality' changes through history, from generation to generation, as cultural attitudes and human knowledge change. An adult, however, has a choice of what to believe and what to reject. So perhaps now is the time for you to re-examine the attitudes and beliefs that form your value system – your statements about the world and the different people within it. In consequence, you will accept that every human being has an equal right to life, choices and care.

ACTIVITY

Think of the clients in your care setting. Select two clients with whom you find it difficult to communicate or accept. Make a special effort, for at least two weeks, to get closer to these clients; create opportunities to talk to them informally and get to know them as people. As you do this, watch out for any prejudices that might prevent you from getting closer to them; for example,

you may have a negative view about the subgroup to which the client belongs, or disapprove about his or her appearance or past history.

Has your general attitude towards these clients changed as a result of your getting to know them as individuals? If not, reflect why and then try again.

Ways of promoting equality

To ensure anti-discriminatory practice and promote equality, you must be willing to:

- examine your attitudes and motives, and become aware of the dangers of your subtle as well as overt behaviour which might discriminate against some clients and colleagues;
- offer the services which your agency provides to all clients who need them;
- inform all clients, irrespective of their backgrounds, about the range of services available to them;
- promote individuals' rights and support clients in making a choice of service, even when this includes their right to reject help;
- respect the rights of clients, their relatives and carers to confidentiality. Inform them of instances when other professionals might need to share information about them, explaining the reasons.

ACTIVITY

1 Get in touch with the two organisations listed below and ask them to send you information on their role in society.

Commission for Racial Equality
Eliot House
10–12 Allington Street
London SW1E 5EH
Tel. 0171 828 7022

Disabled Living Foundation
380–384 Harrow Road
London W9 2HU
Tel. 0171 289 6111

2 When you have done this, think of a situation when you or your clients might need their help or advice.

3 Working with people individually

3.1 Changing roles of care agencies

The implementation of the Community Care Act (see section 1.4) has brought and is still bringing changes to both the structures and the roles of agencies that provide health and social care to clients. The end result of these changes is still to be seen, but the most significant change is in who does what within the wide range of agencies and their staff. So, for example, while some carers and agencies are expected to manage or co-ordinate the care work for an individual client, assess that client's care needs and decide on how the available resources are spent, others might be responsible mainly for providing the actual care.

The two most common ways of working are case management and the key worker system, while the team approach system is less popular.

Case management

One of the major changes has been the introduction of a case management style of working. A case manager – most often a social worker, but sometimes another type of professional – has special responsibility for the care of individual clients. He or she is not the main provider of care and services, but manages both resources and care. This may include responsibilities such as:

- finding individuals who have care needs;
- assessment of the clients' needs;
- planning care: formulating care plans for individual clients, budget planning and monitoring purchasing of care services;
- ensuring that the care needs of clients are met and care plans are implemented;
- being a central point of contact for individual clients;
- co-ordinating, monitoring and reviewing the care provided to the clients by a range of providers from statutory, voluntary or private sectors.

Case managers need not necessarily do all of this, but they are responsible for seeing that it is done.

Key worker system

Under the key worker system, each client is allocated one worker who will be responsible for his or her overall care and care programme. You do not

---

ACTIVITY

Do you have a case manager in your care setting, or have you met one through your work or through your training? If you know one, arrange to meet to discuss exactly what she does. Ask her to talk to you about her case management of the clients whom you already know.

have to be a social worker or a nurse to be a key worker. The main criterion is that you possess the skills and understanding needed to care for the clients for whom you are responsible. Your responsibilities will include:

- contributing to the ongoing assessment of the client's needs, the evaluation of care and the formulation of care plans;
- contributing to the planning and carrying out of the care programme, development and therapeutic activities, and rehabilitation;
- contributing to the health and safety of the client and his environment;
- communicating relevant information to the client, and co-ordinating communication with other professionals (e.g. case conferences);
- involving the client in decision making about his care;
- helping in advocacy, that is acting on the client's behalf or liaising with other advocates.

You will not necessarily be responsible for all of these all the time: the client may participate in care programmes, such as various group activities provided by other workers and agencies.

Even if your agency does not operate a key worker system, the fact that you are a named worker for clients referred to your care setting means that you will still have some, if not all, of the above responsibilities.

Team approach to care

Occasionally agencies use a system where they encourage clients to approach any worker they want, subject to their availability at the time, for specific help. The whole team (all the agency's workers) is then responsible for the care of each client, while each worker is accountable to the team and the manager for the specific task which she or he has undertaken. While this style of working discourages clients' dependency on one worker, some clients might feel threatened and find it unsettling to have so many different workers engaged with them.

Where do you fit in?

Your role is to assist care professionals who have senior positions and probably specialist training. This means that you will be supporting them when asked, irrespective of the job title or position which they hold. So your work could consist of helping social workers, nurses, occupational therapists or home care organisers (for domiciliary care).

Whichever style of working your care setting employs, your supervisor will give you guidance about how you fit into this complex, ever-changing care environment. You will probably also have a written job description.

ACTIVITY

1 Ask your supervisor what system of working is used in your care setting and how it operates. Do this during one of your supervision meetings with her if you have them.

2 Ask for clarification of the roles and responsibilities of different members of your care team, focusing on those aspects of work which might overlap with your own responsibilities.

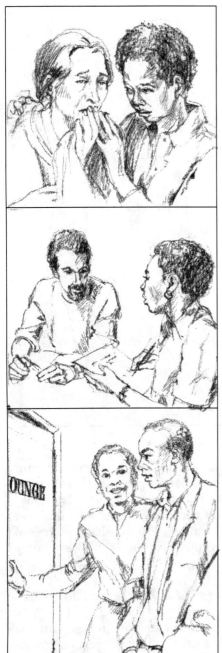

3.2 Professional relationships

What are they?

Relationships are professional when people interact for a clear purpose in a way expected of them within their profession. Such a relationship includes how you:

- present yourself through your personal appearance and demeanour;
- communicate with others;
- fulfil your duties and responsibilities according to your role, your agency's policies and government legislation.

With whom?

You will be expected to have a professional relationship with a wide range of people, including:

- clients;
- clients' families and friends;
- clients' representatives, e.g. advocates (see section 3.8);
- colleagues;
- your supervisor, manager and other superior staff;
- supportive staff employed by your agency, e.g. secretaries, clerks, technicians and information technology workers;
- other professionals and carers, e.g. doctors, nurses, psychologists, psychotherapists and occupational therapists (see section 3.1);
- the general public, e.g. people who enquire about your agency;
- employees of welfare services such as the DSS and housing department.

Knowing your responsibilities and limitations

You can only act professionally if you are fully aware of your responsibilities and know where your responsibility ends.

Caring in mental health demands a wide range of skills and knowledge, from giving emotional support to clients, to helping them with practical, financial and educational needs. You also need to know about services and issues outside your care setting, and to keep up with all the changes within them.

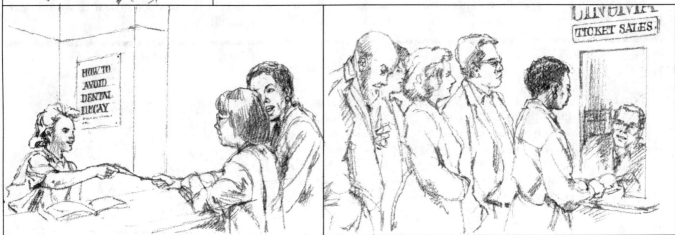

A care worker doing a range of tasks

However, you cannot know and do everything, so acknowledging your limitations is important.

Professional relationships with clients

You may think that the term 'professional relationship' suggests a relationship which is distant, cold or even superficial. While this may be so with some professions, it certainly is not or should not be in a care setting. Mental health care, in particular, needs workers who are sensitive, genuine and warm, and able to understand and sympathise with clients. At the same time, it needs workers who are able to be strict and businesslike when such an attitude is called for. You should be able to say 'No' when your professional judgement tells you to, and to stick to the practices or policy of your organisation despite any protest and adverse emotional reaction you might get from clients – and despite your own emotional attachment to the clients as well.

Relationship boundary

Professional relationships with clients have a boundary – limitations in behaviour – which relates to the degree of your intimacy and personal involvement. This boundary applies to all care settings; it especially concerns sexual relations between a client and a worker. Such a relationship is highly unprofessional, with an implication of abuse of power by the worker. In most cases any socialising outside the work context is also inappropriate.

ACTIVITY

Ask two colleagues to take part in a role play in which you are the worker, one of your colleagues is a client, and the other acts as an observer.

You are the only worker in the centre's drop-in for the remaining 15 minutes of its opening hours. All your colleagues have left the building and gone home.

Your agency has a policy of prohibiting drinking or serving alcoholic drinks on its premises. Ten minutes before the closure, Mary – a client with whom you have an especially good and warm working relationship – comes in. It is her birthday, and she has rushed from the other end of town to get to the centre on time so that you can have a drink with her. Other clients are leaving, which leaves you and Mary alone. 'Only a small drink – no one will ever know', she insists, producing a bottle from her handbag bought especially for the occasion. You remind her of the agency's 'No drinking' policy, but Mary becomes very emotional and at the verge of tears, pleading 'Please, I have no one to have a drink with me on my birthday. You're my only friend.'

1 What do you say to her? What do you do?

2 After the role play, discuss your reasons for the chosen action. Then let the colleagues, beginning with the observer, share their views on how they would deal with a similar situation.

Using your creativity

Each situation which demands your professional judgement and behaviour requires an individual approach. However, you should always aim to treat your clients with warmth and empathy. If you need to say 'No', the client will feel less disappointed if you first acknowledge her need or wish, take time to explain your reasons for refusal, and do this in a way which she is likely to understand and accept. Try to be creative to soften the blow of refusal – which, as in Mary's case (see previous activity), might be received as personal rejection. A sense of humour can help too, especially when you have a good rapport with a client.

Remember that being friendly with clients does not mean being friends, even if they choose to misinterpret your friendliness, which happens when people are very lonely.

Be polite

Being polite towards clients shows respect for them as human beings. One of the effects of social attitudes towards people experiencing mental health difficulties is lack of respect. Saying that someone is 'mad' or 'crazy', even in jest or behind her back, is showing disrespect. Strive to be polite to clients even when they seem to have lost touch with reality, as, for example, when they experience hallucinations (see section 1.2).

Greet clients

Greeting someone or responding when you are being greeted shows a recognition of that individual's existence. It is extremely important to clients' self-esteem.

Listen

Listening to clients when they are speaking to you (see section 3.3) shows politeness and respect. Listening includes paying attention by making eye-contact instead of looking at something or someone else. Listening shows that you are interested in both the client as an individual and what she is saying.

Be tactful

To be tactful you have to be sensitive to the situation you are in and the person's reaction to it. If you sense, for example, that the client's mood swing is making him oversensitive to a particular issue which you are discussing, be careful how you proceed. Ask yourself the following questions.

- Is it important to resolve the issue here and now, or can it be postponed until the client has calmed down?
- Are you politely asking the client to do something, to keep his morning appointment with his doctor, for example, or are you ordering him to do it? The tone and pitch of your voice and your body posture can reveal this.
- When you must be strict or say 'No', are you aware of how the client might feel and how much disappointment that would cause, so that you try to soften the blow? Or do you carry out your work and your 'orders' from your superiors with an air of cold, punitive authority?
- Do you take time to explain things to clients and to make sure that they have understood the reasons why something must or must not be done?

Understand rebellion against authority

Sometimes clients see staff as representatives of an authority against which they wish to rebel. Most of us slip into such attitudes at times, especially when we feel that we lack control of a situation or power over our lives. Understanding that your clients' hostility is not directed at you personally, but against what you represent, might help you deal with such incidents. If you are tactful, and negotiate if necessary, you may avoid a situation which is potentially destructive or upsetting to other clients.

Self-disclosure

When you are in an informal situation with a client with whom you have a good rapport, the client might insist that you reveal some personal information. You might be tempted to oblige her, not only because you wish to please her but also perhaps because you feel a need to unburden some of your personal traumas. Always reflect on what would be appropriate, considering the professional nature of your relationship, regardless of how warm, understanding or special that relationship may be, and regardless of whether or not your colleagues or supervisor would ever get to hear it.

In refusing to give personal information, avoid asking 'Why do you wish to know?' This suggests defensiveness. Instead, you might say 'I don't see how knowing that helps your situation.' In that way you are focusing on the client and her needs – not on yours.

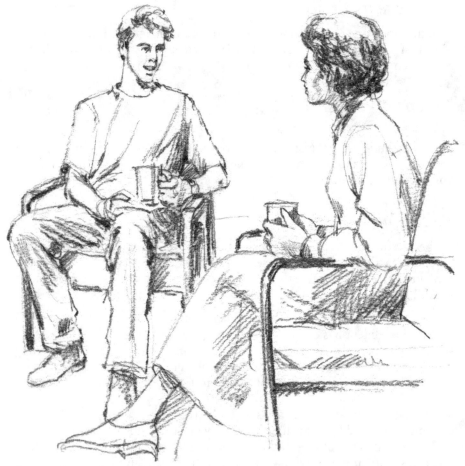

Care worker to client: 'If I start telling you my problems, we'll be here until Christmas!'

Humour can help

In dealing with demands such as sharing personal information, tact is paramount. A sense of humour can sometimes ease the feeling of rejection which the clients might experience when you refuse to answer personal questions.

When dilemmas arise

At times you will be faced with a dilemma about how to act or what to say to clients. Such situations will not always have clearly defined rules on how to proceed. Much will depend on:

ACTIVITY

Consider the following situations with one or more colleagues, working in pairs or in a small group.

1 You find out that you share the same passion for an actor with a client whose company you find enjoyable. The latest film featuring this actor is being shown; all the tickets are sold out well in advance. Unexpectedly your client tells you that he has been given two tickets and wants you to go with him. Will you accept?

2 A client makes a pass at you. What is your reaction?

3 You live in a large town or city and you travel by bus to the day centre where you work. On your way home you meet a client from another borough who has just been attached to your day centre. He chats with you as the bus approaches your stop, and tells you that he lives in a road which is a ten-minute walk from the next bus stop. He is not yet aware that this is also your stop. What do you do?

Discuss your individual suggestions and then ask your supervisor for his or her comments.

- your care setting and its practices;
- the client's level of dependency and the nature of care he is receiving;
- the client's cultural expectations;
- your particular role and your range of skills and knowledge as well as limitations.

Do not give out your address

For your own protection and privacy, you should never give clients your address. In situations where this arises, you will have to be creative. For example, in situation 3 of the previous activity you would be forgiven for telling the client that you are visiting a friend in the area, making sure that you are not followed. Even better, you could miss your stop and get off at the next one.

Do not show favouritism

You may find that you prefer caring for some clients more than others. Their personality, background, disposition and attitude towards you as a carer and person will influence how you feel and think about them. But you must try hard not to allow this to influence the way you conduct yourself in your professional capacity. Showing favouritism, which inevitably gives a message of rejection to others who are excluded, is not professional.

Points to consider in ensuring a professional relationship

The questions below can help you develop and maintain a professional relationship with clients.

- Is your action here in accordance with your professional role?
- Is your professional working relationship with the client going to suffer or improve if you agree to his request?
- What is the best way to reject the client's inappropriate suggestion or demand, without making her feel that you are rejecting her as a person?
- How can you show your professional authority without undermining the client's identity and worth?
- Are your reasons for exerting your authority and control understood by the client, and if not, how do you make sure that they are?
- How will telling the client personal information about yourself help her? If it will not, avoid telling her.
- Are you influenced by your prejudices in your work with clients? If you suspect that you might be, talk to your supervisor.

3.3 Listening and supporting

The ability to listen

Good professional relationships demand good communication skills, which consist of more than just possessing an adequate vocabulary. Of course, it helps if you happen to be a fluent and confident speaker: you may know someone who is really good at this. Yet some people with such a gift hardly ever listen to what others have to say!

How we listen

Your work with clients will not always be carried out in ideal conditions for listening – secluded and quiet surroundings, free from other activities or demands. Neither are you always fully attentive. No one can listen all the time to everything. However, you should aim to recognise when clients need you to listen, and set aside time and a suitable place where you can give them your full attention.

Time to listen

You will find that some of your clients are too impatient to wait for an appointment. They have such a low tolerance of stress and uncertainty that the only way they can cope is to unburden their troubles onto you at the first opportunity. However, if you happen to be on your way elsewhere at the time – a prior arrangement to visit a client, for example – it is better to gently explain this to the client. Give an alternative time whenever possible, or suggest that the client sees another worker who is coming on duty after you. Stopping to listen to the client while you are looking at your watch and thinking about the next job is not going to be productive.

Stick to your priorities

Dropping everything else to give attention to a client every time he or she asks for it is not helpful, because the care setting should provide some learning experience of the world at large. People do not generally drop everything to make someone else their immediate priority. Exceptions to this include emergency situations which require immediate attention.

When is 'here-now' listening a must?

Your instincts should tell you when this is. When you hear a client calling you because another one has just had a fall or has locked herself in the bathroom, for example, you should see to it right away. Less obvious incidents should also alert you.

Examples

1   A client tells you: 'There are lots of sparks coming from my radio as I plug it in, and I want to listen to my favourite programme which starts in five minutes.'

   You will have to do something to ensure the client's safety. Passing on the message to a colleague before you leave, or removing the radio yourself from the client's room for it to be seen by an electrical engineer, might be acceptable courses of action. Any electrical appliance should be removed as soon as the client has pointed out that something might be wrong with it, and marked or labelled 'dangerous'.

2   A client has casually mentioned that she has just swallowed a dozen Paracetamol tablets.

   This must be immediately reported to a doctor. Tell your supervisor first and check about calling an ambulance. Anything involving taking an overdose of medication or swallowing some harmful substance such as bleach should be attended to right away by referring the problem to medical staff.

3   Accidents of any nature which have left someone injured – falls, cuts or anything else which might require your attention or the attention of other professionals – must be attended to directly.

ACTIVITY

Do the following activity over two days.

1 Choose the first opportunity at the end of each working day to note down *how* you listened to two individual clients during that day. Consider the following questions:

- What activity, if any, were you engaged in with each client or someone else at the time?
- How interested were you in what the client was telling you – be honest. Note your interest on a five point scale, where 1 is for 'not interested at all' and 5 is 'very interested indeed'.
- What was the atmosphere around you like? Was it just the two of you in a room, or was the room bustling with clients or other workers? Was there background noise such as music playing or people talking?
- Were you relaxed, agitated, tired, or under pressure and keen to get away?

- Were you thinking of something else at the time, such as the next thing you had to do or other personal thoughts?

2 Note down what, if anything, you did or intended to do about what you heard when listening to each client. This should include:

- telling your supervisor or colleagues your concerns about what the client has told you;
- getting in touch with the client's doctor or family, welfare and other services;
- doing or arranging to do something practical for the client yourself;
- obtaining, via appropriate channels, relevant information for or about the client;
- giving emotional support such as encouragement.

Privacy and quiet

Listening and supporting should be done in a room allocated for this purpose, or in a private area. Clients who live on the premises or use the day centre regularly and so know everyone there may not always expect or wish to go with you to another room. Follow your instincts on such occasions, but offer total privacy whenever possible. Clients who have just come in from outside, if your agency has an 'open door' policy whereby anyone can walk in asking for help, are likely to shy away if you do not offer them privacy.

Listening as support

Listening to a client means paying attention. You can show that you are doing this by using relevant non-verbal communication skills: an 'open' body posture, eye-contact and occasional nodding of the head (see section 2.5). But giving support usually means doing more than listening. As you probably noticed in the last activity, it could involve a course of action or emotional support. Do the next activity to explore what you and your colleagues understand by the term 'support'.

Emotional support

Emotional support can include:

- feeling someone had the time and patience to hear you out;
- being encouraged to express yourself on difficult issues;
- being understood and shown empathy (see overleaf);
- being shown a non-judgemental attitude irrespective of how you think, feel or behave;
- being given a realistic hope at times of despair;
- being offered some other help, when appropriate.

ACTIVITY

Ask two or more colleagues or friends to participate in this informal discussion.

1 Each member in turn should say what it means to her or him to be 'given support' in any aspect of living.

2 Do you think that some of the meanings provided by the group can be applied to the clients in your care setting? If so, which ones?

Empathy and empathic understanding

To feel empathy is to feel with or for clients. But it is not enough just to feel sympathetic towards someone's pain or misfortunes; as a carer you should be able to communicate your fellow-feeling to the client, verbally and non-verbally. This is empathic understanding (see case study below), which is in itself therapeutic as clients feel understood on an emotional level. It represents one of the main ingredients of emotional support.

How to give emotional support

You have probably given your clients emotional support, including empathic understanding, without realising it. Most carers soon learn that, as well as practical caring, less tangible kinds are important as well. In mental health, emotional support is often the basis for all other work with or for clients. The next activity is designed to help you become more aware of what you actually do when you are listening to clients' problems.

> **ACTIVITY**
>
> *1* Read the case study below and then write down which of the care worker's responses helped the client to disclose difficult personal information and which acknowledged the client's feelings.
>
> *2* Has the worker given the client any hopeful responses? If so, are they realistic or not?
>
> *3* In what way, if any, is the care worker's last sentence helpful?

> **CASE STUDY**
>
> *Client*: I had a really difficult time with my parents during my last visit.
>
> 1 *Care worker* (making eye-contact, with an 'open' body posture facing the client): You had a difficult time?
>
> *Client*: Yes. It was worse than last time. I was so upset that I thought of cutting myself off completely. But then, thinking of my mother, I guess I could never do that to her.
>
> 2 *Care worker*: Sounds serious. I wonder what made you feel that way?
>
> *Client*: Well. Er . . .
>
> 3 *Care worker*: Yes?
>
> *Client* (encouraged as the worker looks at him sympathetically and paying full attention): I am sure my father does not want me to visit. He just kept on contradicting me all the time whenever I spoke. (Angrily) And he called me a liar when I told mum about the time he took me with him when he visited his lady friend. I was 12 at the time and knew what he was up to.
>
> 4 *Care worker*: You mean you talked about the past when your father was unfaithful to your mother? (Nod from the client) That must have been difficult.
>
> *Client*: Oh, it was! For my mother especially! But she wanted to know. She insisted I should tell her all I know – so I did. Do you think I did the right thing? (Looking at the worker anxiously) She knows about his other lovers. Perhaps I shouldn't have said about that one?
>
> 5 *Care worker*: You said she asked you to tell her, so you did. Isn't that what she wanted?
>
> *Client*: I guess so. It's just that the confrontation with my father was horrible. If only he would stop behaving like that. Why doesn't she leave him? I don't understand it.

6 *Care worker*: Do you get on better with your mother then?

Client: Oh, yes! I guess I visit mainly because of her. I feel sorry for her, having to put up with my father all these years.

7 *Care worker*: Your mother must appreciate your visits. She must know you care for her.

Client (quite emotional, on the verge of tears): I wish I could do something. I am stuck here with my problems and my mother has to put up with him.

8 *Care worker*: You feel unhappy, maybe even helpless that you can't solve the marriage problems of your parents. Yet, you're doing the best you can at the moment. By being here you are recovering from your own emotional setback, and the stronger you get, the more support you'll be able to give your mother. She knows you care for her, which must bring her some comfort. And you visit home regularly despite everything.

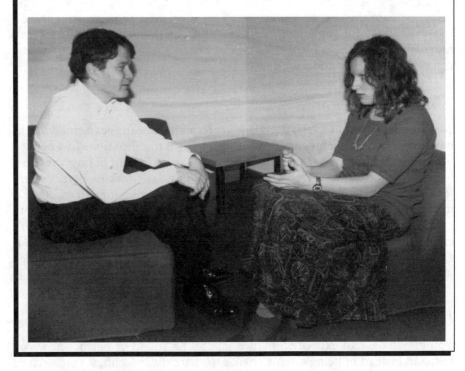

Appropriate responses

Acknowledging the client's feelings is one of the most helpful ways of giving emotional support. In the previous case study, some acknowledgement of how the client feels is shown by the worker's responses 1, 2, 4 and 8. Note that in response 1, the worker repeats the *key words* used by the client, with an inflection to show a questioning tone. Initially the client is vague; in response 2 the worker encourages and prompts him to use concrete examples of what has happened.

Response 3 ('Yes?') is an *encourager*, and an example of what is known as a 'minimal response'. Other minimal responses include head nodding, smiling or other facial expressions, and simple sounds. Their purpose is to show that you are listening and to encourage the client to continue with minimal interruption from you.

The worker expresses understanding of how the client feels (empathy) in response 7. Notice how after she says 'She must know you care for her', the client becomes emotional. It seems that the worker has touched upon a sensitive issue here – how much the client cares for his mother. This is an example of accurate empathy. We know that it is accurate from the client's next sentence – 'I wish I could do something' – and from his general comments about his mother and father throughout.

In the final response the worker gives a summary of what the client expressed earlier, thereby, again, acknowledging his feelings. This is *pacing*, when the feelings expressed by the client, through words or other means, are verbalised by the worker. The second sentence in 8, however, marks the beginning of the worker *leading* the client towards a more hopeful position. Is the third sentence here realistic? Clearly it is, because it states the reality of the situation: the client's dependence on the mental health centre will help him get better and emotionally stronger. He will only be able to help his mother more if he helps himself first. By pointing out the helpful things he is already doing – home visits, showing his mother he cares for her – the worker helps increase the client's self-esteem. This is called a *positive asset search*: the carer looks for something positive in the client and communicates it to him. This should help lift the feelings of helplessness expressed earlier and can become a foundation for new hope.

A note of caution

Not all interaction in which the client expresses sad feelings can end with the worker giving a hopeful comment. It depends on the situation. Just being a listener and giving verbal and non-verbal acknowledgement of how the client feels might be sufficient at times. For example, at times of bereavement (discussed in Chapter 5), giving the clients hope can be inappropriate if it minimises the impact of the loss. The client must be given the opportunity to grieve before any hopeful comments are made. Staying with the client emotionally – that is, not rushing to change the painful or unpleasant emotions expressed at the time to more hopeful ones – is an art which is much needed in everyday life and in caring.

Listen – do not advise

You may have had experiences when you told a friend or partner how you felt, and instead of being given a chance to share those feelings, you received unwanted and inappropriate advice. Consider the following:

- 'Don't worry.' (Who can stop worrying by simply being told not to?)
- 'It's not as bad as you feel.' (Only you can know that. You are an individual and have a right to feel in your own way and at your own intensity.)
- 'You shouldn't feel that way because . . .' (There is no 'should' about how you feel; you just feel. Again, you want acceptance of your emotions.)
- 'Everyone feels like that sometimes.' (Is this really helping you right now? It can minimise what you are feeling; you are not 'everyone'!)
- 'A similar thing happened to me . . .' (A story follows and the focus is shifted, so you find yourself having to listen to someone else's past misfortune at a time when you need support for your own current troubles.)

Unhelpful comments or advice are given by people who feel uncomfortable not knowing what to do or say to help you. They tell you how you should feel with the best of intentions. It might make them feel better, but often makes you feel worse.

In your work with clients, try to recognise such tendencies in yourself and, instead, become a truly supportive listener.

Listen

When I ask you to listen to me
and you start giving me advice
you have not done what I have asked.

When I ask you to listen to me
and you begin to tell me why I shouldn't feel that way
you are trampling on my feelings.

When I ask you to listen to me
and you feel you have to do something to solve my problem
then you have failed me, strange as it may seem.

Listen! All I ask for is that you listen
not talk or do – just hear me.
Advice is cheap: ten cents will get you both
Dear Abby and Billy Graham in the same newspaper
and I can do for myself: I am not helpless.
Maybe discouraged and faltering, but not helpless.

When you do something for me that I can and need to do
for myself, you contribute to my fear and weakness.
But when you accept as a single fact
that I do feel what I feel
no matter how irrational, then I can quit
trying to convince you and get about the business
of understanding what's behind
this irrational feeling.
And when tact is clear, the answers are obvious,
and I don't need advice.
Irrational feelings make sense when we understand
what's behind them.

Perhaps that's why prayers work sometimes for some people
because God is mute, and he doesn't give advice or
try to fix things. 'They' just listen and let you
work it out for yourself.

So please listen and just hear me. And if you want to
talk, wait a minute for your turn: and
I'll listen to you.

Anonymous

3.4 Dealing with problems in communication

Communication between clients and workers, or between one client and another, does not always run smoothly. This section describes a range of problems and suggests how you might deal with them. By helping clients to overcome communication difficulties you will also help them to make relationships with others, because relationships cannot exist or last without adequate communication.

Language barriers

Communication can be difficult when the client's first language is not English, or when his level of understanding is insufficient for the complex emotional, psychological and social issues of mental health. To minimise this, you and your care team should be as clear as possible about the client's race and culture, country of birth, number of years in this country, and age or gender, which can give you clues about the possibility of a language barrier.

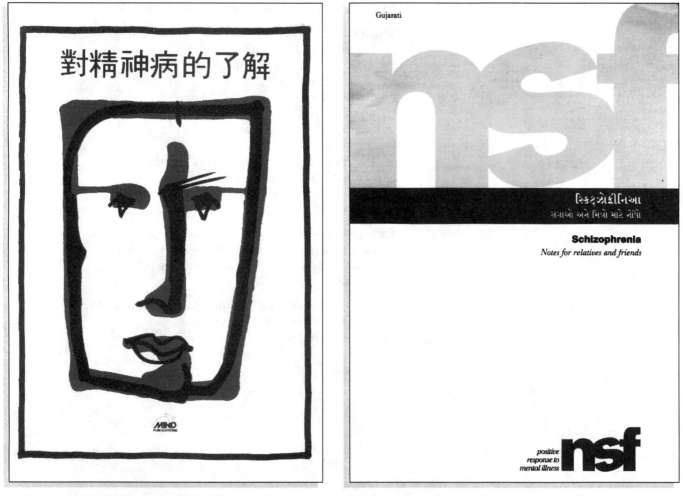

Leaflets are available in languages other than English
(a) Understanding mental illness (Cantonese)   *(b) Notes on schizophrenia (Gujarati)*

Using interpreters

Your senior colleagues can give you advice about the approach used by your organisation for cases when language might be a problem. Some agencies have contact with a pool of interpreters which they employ on such occasions. Make sure that the interpreter speaks the same dialect as the client. When this is not possible family members may be used, but avoid using the client's child because the problem might be too personal or too complex. If these options are not available or not adequate for the kind of work you are to undertake with the client, it might be better to refer the client to another agency with the proper resources.

Non-verbal language

As was pointed out in section 2.6, there are some cultural differences in the use and interpretation of body language.

CASE STUDY

Jo comes from a non-British Black culture where it is acceptable to sit quite close to the person you are speaking to and touch him or her occasionally as a way of stressing certain words. He is a newcomer to a day centre where almost all clients and staff are White British, but this does not bother him as he is friendly, outgoing and enjoys meeting all sorts of people. However, his non-verbal behaviour soon becomes a problem – others find Jo too familiar and some clients feel threatened. Those of the opposite sex misinterpret Jo's habit of touching as a sexual overture. They complain to staff and Jo gets reprimanded. After several such incidents, Jo feels rejected and abruptly breaks all contact with the centre.

Jo's experience suggests one of the reasons why Black clients are under-represented in mental health care settings. Care professionals, and the White British culture as a whole, currently have a poor understanding of the non-verbal communication of others.

A care worker from another culture

If you are a care worker from a culture whose non-verbal language is different from the majority of your clients, take care to avoid those aspects – such as touching or sitting too close – which they might find threatening. This means you will have to modify your gestures to fit in with those around you. This is not easy because most of our non-verbal communication is automatic and unconscious, so you will need to bring your body movement under conscious control.

Help to educate your colleagues

The above suggestion does not imply that you should abandon the traditions of your cultural origin. Seek an opportunity to introduce this topic to both your colleagues and clients, and help them understand such cultural differences. Educating them will help to ensure that misunderstandings such as Jo's do not happen in the future.

Equality in caring

For clients from other cultures, such as Black, French or Spanish, a White British worker's physical distance and non-expressive body language might be interpreted as rejection, even hostility, making them feel even more isolated. The principle of equality in caring, which includes clients' personal beliefs about how they should be cared for, demands flexibility from the majority culture's care workers as well. This is a challenging thought, and some organisations are beginning to see value in placing their staff on training courses designed for multicultural awareness.

Limited sensory ability

When clients have limited sensory ability, such as visual and hearing difficulties, they might use sign language, communication by touch, or hearing aids. An interpreter will be needed if a client uses sign language or a touch method of communication. Make sure you follow the procedure of your agency and employ an interpreter who understands the issue of confidentiality.

Hearing aids

If a client uses a hearing aid, check that it is properly inserted and switched on. A high-pitched sound is usually a sign that adjustment is necessary – the client should know how to do this.

If you notice that a client who is using his hearing aid correctly still has difficulty in hearing, alert your supervisor: the client may need to visit a hearing specialist or occupational therapist for reassessment.

A *worker's hearing*

Occasionally, a worker might also have difficulty in hearing, not realising that this could be a sign of hearing impairment. Make sure that you have heard what a client said; there is no harm in asking a client to speak louder or repeat himself. Have your hearing checked if you suspect a problem.

Psycho-social problems in communicating

Some people find it difficult to communicate when they are in a group or with strangers. We might say that they lack social skills. There are evening classes or courses run by adult and community education centres for this sort of problem. Assertiveness courses, where people are taught by role play how to say what they think, feel and want, could also be run within a care agency.

Help clients to communicate

If you notice that a new residential client spends too much time in her room or sits in a corner of the lounge avoiding social contact with others, approach her slowly and gradually establish an informal relationship first. Sit next to the client, after asking for permission to do so, make eye-contact and smile before speaking. You could start by looking for some common ground in order to share a little about yourself. Choose neutral subjects initially, such as what clothes, colours, food, sports or seasons of the year you like best, to

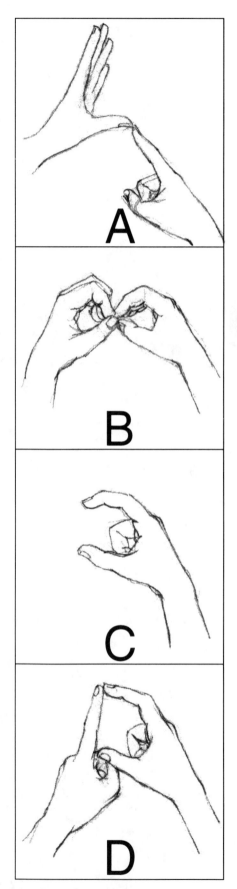

Sign language: letters A, B, C and D

ACTIVITY

1 Ask a senior colleague to discuss with you three recent incidents that took place in your care setting when clients' mental distress caused communication difficulties.

2 Learn how the worker managed, or why he or she did not succeed, to communicate with each client under such conditions.

3 Generate ideas on how you can improve your communication with clients in similar situations in the future.

encourage the client to speak to you and come out of her shell. If you are the key worker for such a client, you may have to spend longer establishing a rapport before you go on to do other practical or social tasks.

Difficulties in communication related to mental distress

Sometimes a phobia of other people could be the cause of a client avoiding the company of others. Clients suffering from this should have fewer workers involved with their care: perhaps just one or two whom they can trust.

Mood fluctuations

When clients experience elation during episodes of mania in manic depression, their communication may become illogical, erratic and confused. It is also difficult to communicate with someone during episodes of deep depression, when everything, including the effort to communicate, is viewed by the sufferer as pointless and futile. Sometimes depression is replaced by aggression. You might find it even more difficult to communicate with clients who, during relapse, are experiencing an episode of delusion.

Accept clients' symptoms

You will have to learn to accept clients' mental health symptoms and mood changes, and the confusing or disruptive communication that can result. Learn how to respond in each situation; every client's way of coping is unique. As you get to know individual clients better, you will learn how they are likely to react during a relapse.

Isolation of clients

Communication problems related to mental health can cause great distress to other clients. Sometimes isolating disruptive clients – by asking them to leave the room – is the only way to avoid this. Make sure that you explain why he or she is being isolated. However, you should never isolate clients merely because you find them tiresome or can't be bothered to make an extra effort to communicate with them. Many symptoms of mental heath difficulties are challenging, and as a care worker you should strive to help clients overcome them – never punish the victim of these symptoms.

Questioning clients

Mental health clients, perhaps more than other client groups, are questioned by an army of professionals: doctors, psychiatrists, nurses, housing department staff, welfare department officials, police officers, social workers, occupational therapists, and so on. It is not surprising that some have become wary of any professional who asks questions.

Control your curiosity

You should avoid asking questions out of curiosity. Ask yourself whether the question you wish to ask could provide answers which will, in some way, help you care for the client. If it won't, don't ask it.

'Closed' and 'open' questions

A closed question generates a limited set of answers, usually 'yes' or 'no'. An open question, however, can generate a wide range of answers. Here are some examples for you to consider:

Closed:

- Did you make an appointment with your doctor?
- Do you feel angry when you do not get a reply from your friend?
- Have you got two hours free this week?

Open:

- What have you done about your injury?
- How do you feel when you do not get a reply from your friend?
- In what way do you find that interesting?

ACTIVITY

Read the examples of 'closed' and 'open' questions and write down which type of question you would prefer to use for your clients and why.

Which kind of questions should you ask?

The type of questions you use will depend on what you wish to know. Consider the previous examples. Do you want to know exactly whether or not the client made an appointment to see her doctor about the injury, or are you interested in what she has done about the injury, including other possibilities such as putting a bandage on it herself? As you can see, the answer to an open question might be too vague if you need specific information to confirm whether or not something is true.

Use open questions for emotions

When the topic in question might include a range of answers, such as those to do with the client's inner world – feelings, attitudes, thoughts and perceptions – it is far better to ask open questions. Using a closed question would involve guessing or assuming what the client feels or thinks, and you have a good chance of getting it wrong. You also have a greater chance of being misled, because clients often wish to agree with the carer in order to be accepted and liked. You might even find that the client becomes defensive when you ask closed questions, perhaps because she is not ready to trust you.

Consider an open question such as 'How do you feel about . . .?' You can see that it allows a range of feelings and explanations to be voiced. By not limiting the answers, you are giving the client freedom and permission to confide in you. As well as giving you more information, it can be therapeutic for the client.

Therapeutic communication

Other verbal skills which will help you give emotional support to clients include reflecting, paraphrasing and summarising. We will look at each of these in turn.

Reflecting

One way of checking if you have understood what the client has told you is by repeating what he said; if you can do this in slightly different words, while using the same key words (see section 3.3), so much the better. Repeating or reflecting to the client what he or she has just told you is a technique that was first employed in client-centred therapy (see Chapter 1), although other approaches also use it.

Example

Client: I am so mad at my daughter for getting engaged to Steve.

Care worker: You're angry with her because of her engagement to Steve.

Reflecting may seem to you to be a parrot-like repetition of what the client says. However, for a client who is distressed and willing to share his distress with a helper, it is a way of communicating that he has been heard and that the carer is patient – not rushing to ask for self-disclosure. It also has a therapeutic impact. By hearing from the carer what he has just expressed, the client is given time to take in the full personal meaning of his revelation. Alternatively, he is given a chance to think again about what he has said, to examine its accuracy and qualify it further.

Paraphrasing

Paraphrasing is similar to reflection, but you use different words to express what the client has told you. Make sure that you use words which are familiar and meaningful to the client.

Example

Client: My brother got so depressed over his wife leaving him that he had to see his doctor to get sleeping tablets. I had an argument with his wife before she left and told her she wasn't good enough for him. Seeing him in such a state I . . . I feel as if I caused her to leave him.

Care worker: Hum . . . You feel that somehow you're to blame for your brother's marriage break-up and its effects on him.

By paraphrasing, you are:

- showing that you are listening;
- checking with the client that you have heard him correctly;
- asking the client to validate his expressed feelings (by raising your voice at the end of the repeated sentence).

As in reflecting, the client has a chance to re-examine his stated feelings or attitudes, and then to qualify them or reveal more.

Summarising

A summary of the important points which the client and the worker have been talking about can be used at appropriate points in the conversation. For instance, you may want to briefly summarise the key points after the client has been speaking for five minutes or more, going into some detail. You should always summarise at or towards the end of a session with the client. Aim to stress the main problem discussed, giving the client the chance to correct you if you misunderstood him. Then you can use the summary to draw a conclusion. This could be emotionally supportive (see section 3.3) or suggest further action to be taken either by yourself or the client, depending on the nature of the problem.

How successful are you in helping clients to communicate?

You will, undoubtedly, feel pleasure every time you manage to encourage a client to communicate – especially someone for whom it is difficult – or when you succeed in getting the co-operation of a client who is difficult to manage due to a mental health relapse. But there will be times when difficulties in communicating with clients persist, no matter what you try.

If you carry out the activity above, you might be successful in helping clients to communicate with others by first talking with you. On the other hand, you might find that they have not changed at all despite your efforts. Whatever the outcome, you will have a better understanding of their problems in communicating with others, and so have a greater appreciation of this life skill which most of us take for granted.

3.5 Helping clients to use local services

Many clients need help from care workers in carrying out the day-to-day tasks of everyday living, which involve using a range of services in the locality and sometimes elsewhere. You therefore need to know what is offered in your area, by whom, where, and how it can be obtained.

Know about local services

Whether you work in a day centre or residential home, or are helping clients in their own homes, you need to know about health and welfare services which the clients might need.

ACTIVITY

Write down the local addresses of the following agencies:

- general practitioner (GP);
- Department of Social Security (DSS);
- Housing Benefit office;
- housing department;
- social services department;
- hostels for homeless people;
- women's refuge centre;
- hospitals: psychiatric, general, casualty departments;
- community psychiatric nurse (CPN);
- occupational therapist;
- psychotherapist, psychologist;
- ophthalmic practitioner or eye medical centre;
- home help.

When possible, add a phone number and the name of the person whom your care setting usually contacts. You could set these in a chart entitled *Local services network: health and welfare*.

Homeless clients

Homelessness is a growing problem. It has been estimated that about 50 per cent of homeless people experience mental distress (*Access to Health*, 1992). Yet this same research found that 'if some individuals with mental health problems receive several nights of sleep, an adequate diet and warm social contact, some of their symptoms may subside'. Besides, having a home is one of the basic human needs (see Maslow's hierarchy of needs, section 1.3).

How you can help

Your organisation may hold an 'open door' policy so that anyone can walk in off the street to make enquiries, refer themselves for specific help, or just sit in the drop-in centre and have a cup of tea. In this situation, your first aim as a worker is to welcome the newcomer and see if you can be of help. Homeless people with mental health problems may try to avoid contact with a worker, and may come to the centre purely for warmth, tea or companionship. Their wish to live outside the 'system' may override their need for a home, welfare services and social care. You therefore have to be careful how you approach a client who lives on the streets. Be tactful; try to establish a rapport with these individuals so that you can find out, informally, about their whereabouts, living style and needs.

If a newcomer seeks help from you in finding accommodation, consult your senior colleagues. However, you should be aware of the housing and accommodation services for the homeless in your area and know how to contact them to find out about the availability of places – look in your 'useful addresses resource file'. When someone accepts your help in finding accommodation, he or she may also learn to trust you for further help in the future, such as registering with a doctor or receiving other forms of mental health treatment if necessary.

Welfare benefits

You should know about the main benefits available within the health and welfare system. Most of your clients will qualify for at least one. The amount of entitlement depends on their age, savings and other individual circumstances – you will need to check with the department in question.

ACTIVITY

1 Pick up leaflets from a post office or DSS office on the benefits and financial help for:

- unemployed people;
- people who are sick;
- people with severe disabilities;
- people who need help paying rent and Council Tax.

2 Study the leaflets. If you do not understand anything about a particular benefit, ring the local DSS office and ask for an explanation. See the end of this section for further sources of information on benefits.

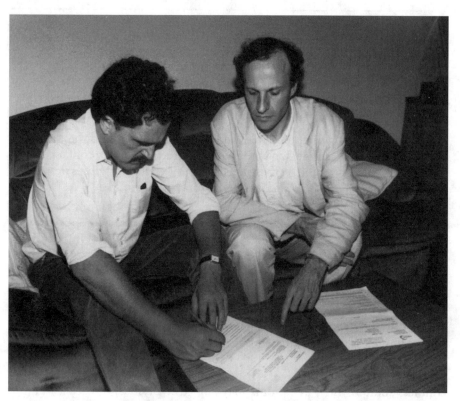

A client and carer working together

Helping clients to apply for benefits

You might have to do this for clients with higher levels of dependency. Long forms can be confusing and even threatening to a client who has just left hospital or has never had to depend on benefits. Applying for help is a stressful and sometimes demoralising event, not least because of social attitudes, so take care to give the clients encouragement and support. When necessary, ring or visit the DSS to help answer questions, or to pursue clients' claims if there are delays.

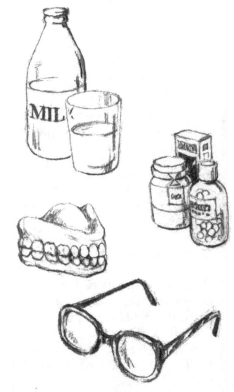

> ### ACTIVITY
>
> *1* Visit your local DSS office and get information leaflets on:
>
> - loans for people in emergencies;
> - grants to help people, such as those with disabilities, to live independently in their homes;
> - loans to help with homemaking and paying bills.
>
> *2* Find out about the eligibility criteria. Talk to a benefit officer if you need more information.

Other services and facilities for clients

You should always ensure that your clients have somewhere to live and receive the benefits to which they are entitled – this is essential. But clients, like other citizens, need to use a range of facilities for their social welfare – in forming

Available on the NHS

and maintaining relationships, personal development, education and training, religious practices, or recreation and sport.

Useful addresses resource file

Your care setting should have a resource file which contains addresses of relevant services and facilities listed in alphabetical order. This supplements the leaflets and brochures produced by agencies which give more general information.

Headings and subheadings for your resource file might look something like this:

A
AIDS
Counselling
Local self-help group
Residential home

Alcoholism
AA
ALANON
Information and counselling

Alzheimer's disease
Counselling for carers
Information
Self-help for carers

Anxiety and phobias
Agoraphobia self-support group
Anxiety management group
Individual counselling
Yoga and meditation group

B
Benefits guide
General enquiries office; Citizen's Advice Bureau (CAB)
Housing Benefit
Invalidity Benefit

Bereavement
Cruse (bereavement counselling): local contact office
And so on . . .

For each entry you would need to know the agency's address and telephone number. You might also include an outline of what each organisation offers, for whom, and the hours when help can be sought. Make sure that it is kept up to date.

ACTIVITY

Draw up a list for your locality, giving the location of the facilities and services named below:

- library;
- post office;
- banks and building societies;
- places of worship: churches, mosques and synagogues;
- adult education centres;

- nurseries and crèches;
- sports centres;
- cinemas and theatres;
- supermarkets and markets;
- parks.

If some of the services are not available in your immediate locality, find out the nearest place where they exist.

Further reading

★   Access to Health has published papers and reports on homelessness and mental health, such as *Mental Health Problems of Homeless People* and *Community Care Plans: A Checklist of the Needs of Homeless People*. Details can be obtained from 32 Chapter Street, London SW1P 4NX. Tel. 0171 233 6599.

★   *Welfare Services* (1993) by Pat Young, part of the *Macmillan Caring Series* published by Macmillan Press, is a level 3 NVQ/SVQ text which focuses on general health and welfare provision.

3.6   Helping clients with living skills

Physical, psychological and social levels of care

Working with clients individually involves caring on several levels: psychological or emotional, social, and physical. The amount of time you spend on each of these during your working day will depend on your care setting and the clients – their age, health and ability to care for themselves. For example, your duties will include more physical or nursing care if you work in a residential home for elderly people with mental health problems or a home for people who have physical disabilities. Nursing staff, including nursing assistants or care assistants, are preferable to social care staff for such clients. You may not have much choice about the kind of care you provide if you care for your partner or a member of your family; ensure that you seek advice and help from professionals for tasks which you find difficult or when you are not sure how to proceed.

Highly dependent clients

This workbook is for care workers, trainees and other carers working with adults of all ages who will, by and large, be capable of self-care – though sometimes with encouragement and guidance from the carer. If you work with clients who need greater assistance in self-care, consult the literature and organisations referred to at the end of this section.

Practical assistance

If you work in a residential care setting for clients with high levels of dependency, or in the home of such a client, you may be expected to provide assistance with a range of practical tasks, such as bathing and dressing. Your employer must provide training on correct lifting techniques if you work with clients who have restricted mobility.

Assessment of mobility

Clients whose physical movement and disability prevent them from doing things for themselves should be assessed by an occupational therapist.

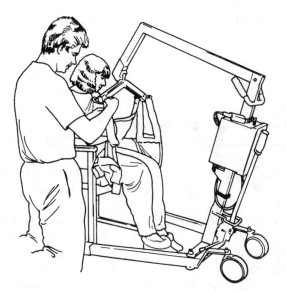

When lifting, use a hoist whenever possible

ACTIVITY

1   Ask the Disabled Living Foundation (see Appendix 2) to send you leaflets and details of information regarding the mobility and personal care of people with physical disabilities.

2   Making sure you have the support of your colleagues and supervisor, arrange a visit by a physiotherapist, occupational therapist or nurse who specialises in caring for people with limited mobility. Prepare questions regarding aspects of personal care of clients which you are unsure about and ask the professional to give you a practical demonstration, for example how to lift a client who is paralysed down one side of the body.

Respect for privacy and dignity

The privacy and dignity of clients who need help with bathing and dressing will suffer, so be sensitive to their needs. Whenever possible, a staff member of the same gender as the client should assist with tasks of personal hygiene. Only stay with a client in a bathroom or bedroom when absolutely necessary for their safety and assistance.

Individual choice

Respect the client's choice of clothes, hairstyle, and other aspects of appearance and cleanliness which are an expression of that client's preference, culture or religion. For example, a Sikh man's hair must not be cut and is covered with a turban, unless the client wishes otherwise; a devout Moslem will need access to water to wash before each prayer.

Food preparation

If your duties involve food preparation, you will need to follow health and safety procedures and guidelines regarding food hygiene. Your training in food hygiene should reflect local requirements. Below are some general guidelines:

- Always wash your hands before and after handling food. Remember that you are a role model for your clients, so you must set a good example. If your or the client's hands have broken skin or cuts, place a waterproof plaster over them and use rubber gloves to avoid direct contact with food, for example when chopping vegetables.
- All those who are involved in food preparation and serving should keep their hair tidy and wear protective clothing such as an apron.
- No smoking should be allowed in the area where food is being prepared.
- All surfaces where you prepare food should be wiped clean before and after use.
- You should observe health and safety procedures when you store food, both cooked and uncooked, taking care to avoid cross-contamination. For example, wrap the food properly and store cooked and uncooked food on different shelves.
- Mark dates on all stored food. The 'use by' dates on manufacturers' labels should be strictly observed.
- If there are clients who are known for attempting self-harm or for harming others, all sharp objects such as knives and scissors should be kept out of reach – but never assume that all people with mental health problems act in such a way.
- When clients with a high level of dependency are using the kitchen for meal preparation, adequate staff supervision should be provided.

Budgeting

If your care setting operates a system by which clients contribute directly from their income (welfare, sickness, invalidity or other sources) towards their lodgings and keep, you may have to help them with or supervise their financial management.

Be tactful when you discuss money with clients. In some cases it is necessary to take money to pay bills and only give the client a personal allowance, but this takes away the individual's control over his or her own life and does not help towards independence. Such a procedure should be viewed only as a temporary solution until the client relearns how to manage a personal budget.

ACTIVITY

1 Arrange to meet one or two clients who cannot manage their budget alone.

2 Draw up a budgeting plan or chart to be filled in during your discussion with the clients. The entries on the chart should reflect each client's individual circumstances. Add columns for when, how and where the payments are to be made (see example on the opposite page).

3 Get each client to agree on a trial period for this budgeting care plan. Set a date to review the results, for example three months later, and record it in your diary.

4 Write down your observations on how the clients are managing during the trial period. You might, for example, record that the client borrowed some money from another client or lent someone some money. Did she get it back? Perhaps she finds it difficult to say 'no' and therefore lends money to clients who are unable to repay the debt.

5 On the review day, discuss how the budgeting went. If the client managed very well, you might like to suggest that she takes more responsibility for handling her own money – larger amounts, for example.

Client's budgeting plan
(based on one month of living in a supported housing association flat)

Name: Date: Review date:

Income and benefits – type:

Total: £–

Outgoing	When due	How paid	Where/what is included
rent: £–	1st of each month	Housing Benefit giro, fortnightly	directly to landlord
water rates: £–	11th of each month	monthly instalment of £–	at the post office, from the savings account
electricity: £– (approx.)	quarterly, next bill due –	from the deposit account	–
food: £–	shopping 2 × per week, Monday and Friday	out of the food allowance allocated at £–	leave money for snacks at the centre
leisure and sundry: £–	as required	weekly spending money £–	include personal hygiene and leisure

ACTIVITY

1 Find out which everyday living skills could be improved for three of your clients: one of high, one of medium, and one of low dependency.

2 Discuss with your supervisor and clients the best ways in which they can be helped to acquire the skills. For example, a client who spends his money on crisps and chocolate, rather than shopping for food that provides an adequate diet, might need to be educated about healthy food before being taught how to prepare simple, nutritious meals.

3 Will this be individual work in which you or another worker, perhaps a dietician, teach the client, or is there a group which the client could join?

Further reading

★ It is now a legal requirement for employers to provide guidance on correct handling techniques. You can, however, save yourself from back injuries (a common outcome of incorrect lifting) by following the guidance set out in the booklet *Are you at risk?* by Janet Daws and Brenda Wright. This is available from Euromed Communications, The Old Surgery, Liphook Road, Haslemere, Surrey GU27 1NL.

★ *Moving and Lifting for Carers* by Martin Hutchinson and Rosemary Rodgers, published in 1991 by Woodhead-Faulkner, is another useful publication.

★ Personal care of clients is covered in more detail in *Caring for People: A Workbook for Care Workers* by Stuart Sillars. This NVQ/SVQ level 2 text is part of the *Macmillan Caring Series* published by Macmillan Press in 1992.

3.7 Contributing to the client's health and safety

Maintaining clients' health and safety depends on many things within a care setting, as well as on many care professionals outside it. Your contribution to this will vary, depending on your duties, your role, and the levels of your clients' dependency.

Appointments with health professionals

Clients who experience a lot of stress and mood fluctuations or are too often self-occupied can easily forget important appointments, such as visits to a GP to discuss medication effects or psychotherapy/counselling sessions. You should remind them of these appointments whenever possible.

Medication

If yours is a residential care setting for clients who have to take medication and who might either forget or take too many tablets in one go, your agency might have a plan whereby care workers have to ensure that all goes well. Your supervisor will explain how your agency deals with medication.

- Learn the most important side effects (see section 1.2). Such knowledge will enable you to inform the client's doctor if the client complains or you notice familiar signs.
- Encourage clients to keep their appointments at depot clinics (see section 1.2) if they are prescribed depot injections.

Infectious diseases

All carers, especially those in a residential setting, should be educated on the right way of carrying out tasks to minimise the risk of spreading infection. This includes HIV/AIDS, hepatitis B and TB.

ACTIVITY

You can either do this test of your knowledge alone, or as a group discussion with your colleagues.

Write down in note form and in three separate columns – one for each viral infection – all the information you know about HIV/AIDS, hepatitis B and TB. In particular, consider the following questions:

- How can the virus be spread?
- What should you and others do to prevent this from happening?
- Which groups or individuals are most likely to be at risk?
- Where and how can you get more information on the virus? Your local doctor's surgery might be a good start.

TO THINK ABOUT

Hepatitis B is spread in the same way as HIV and sometimes with a smaller amount of bodily fluids; it can be as fatal, yet people fear 'catching' HIV/AIDS more than hepatitis B. Why?

ACTIVITY

1 Find out what information about HIV/AIDS is available for the clients in your care setting. For example:

- Do you have a regular supply of leaflets with the basic facts explained? (You can obtain these from a doctor's surgery or from larger chemists.)
- Is this information available in all the languages which are spoken in your locality?

2 Discuss with your supervisor and colleagues ways of educating clients about HIV/AIDS. For example, you might wish to invite an expert, such as a local GP or HIV counsellor, to give a talk.

ACTIVITY

1 Find out about the procedure for keeping written records of accidents or incidents in your care setting (the latter relates to, for example, when one client abuses another client or a carer).

2 Consider why you should make entries of such happenings promptly. Give at least two reasons.

ACTIVITY

Find out about a client in your care setting who has special dietary needs. It might be a low cholesterol diet for those prone to coronary disease, or a diet which a doctor prescribes to avoid the side effects of some medication. How would you ensure that the client follows the prescribed diet?

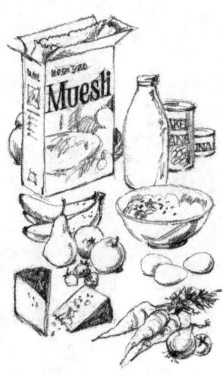

The right diet is an important part of health care

Precautions

Your duty as a care worker is to do all you can to prevent the spread of infection, whether for your clients', colleagues' or your own health. To ensure that you take precautions all the time, you should assume that everyone is or might be HIV positive or infected with hepatitis B.

- Make sure that the first aid box in your care setting always contains rubber gloves.
- Wear rubber gloves whenever you are in a situation where blood or other bodily fluids from another person can, by accident, get mixed with yours. For example, you should wear surgical gloves if you are applying a bandage to someone who has accidentally cut herself because you might have a scratch on your hands even without being aware of it.
- Check your agency's policy for protecting carers against hepatitis B – you might need to be vaccinated.

Prevention of accidents

To help prevent accidents in your care setting, you must strive to keep your environment safe at all times. For example, check that a room where clients meet for a group activity is free from any hazards such as faulty appliances, equipment which needs handling with special care, or dangerous chemical substances.

Follow the health and safety procedures at work as prescribed by your employer; ask to know more about those which you are not sure of. Teach clients how to follow the safety procedures too.

Record keeping

To comply with the Health and Safety at Work Act 1974, you must report anything which adversely affects health and safety at work. It is important to record all accidents promptly and according to the procedure adopted by your agency. If you write up an accident or incident as soon as possible, you are likely to make a more accurate report and so prevent confusion or misrepresentation. If you happen to be absent from work following the accident, your colleagues will know the facts from your report. This may help them deal with any effects which the accident had on the clients or the environment.

Diet

Always support clients in following a diet prescribed by a dietician or their doctor. If your agency provides food, make sure it includes items that such clients need.

Know where your responsibility ends

If you try to do everything – even tasks which you are not qualified or expected to do – you will endanger your own health and safety or that of those you care for, perhaps even both. You must recognise when someone needs specialised or intensive assistance. Talk to senior colleagues whenever in doubt.

3.8 Contributing to the client's advocacy

You might be a passionate believer in equality, but the fact that clients come to your agency for help, often during the most difficult times of their lives, is a clear indication of who has the greater power. Care professionals can give or withhold help and decide on the type of assistance, where it is to be given and by whom; they can delay, refuse or change the course of a care plan according to their professional judgement or prejudices.

TO THINK ABOUT

Think about why a client might need an advocate.

The rights of clients

The above picture is not complete, yet it shows how some clients experience care. Clients have a right to receive the care they need and in the way they choose, while care professionals have a duty to ensure that everyone gets what they are entitled to. This is why legislation exists, so that the clients' rights are safeguarded. But, you may argue, clients still depend on workers to interpret legislation and put the guidelines into practice. No matter how you look at it, clients may still feel that they lack power. This is why you should make a conscious effort to seek the clients' involvement in planning and executing any aspect of their care.

Advocacy

Advocacy helps to ensure that people who are cared for get what they are entitled to and that they, their rights and their property are not abused. There are two types of advocacy: citizen advocacy, when another person acts on behalf of a client, and self-advocacy, when clients do it for themselves, usually by joining together to form a self-advocacy group for mutual support.

CASE STUDY

Sophie and Donald, both in their 30s, met on a psychiatric ward where their admission due to mental health distress coincided on several occasions during a period of two years. They always got on extremely well, comforting and helping each other during crises. Their friendship soon developed further and they continued to meet while living in the community. A year later they became engaged, despite strong opposition from both families.

When finally the couple set a date for their wedding, pressure from their parents to break off the engagement became unbearable. Sophie and Donald therefore asked their key workers to act as advocates, to help persuade their parents to respect their wishes and attend the wedding.

What do advocates do?

This will depend on the problem and on each agency's policy. In the example of Sophie and Donald (see above case study), the care workers met to discuss a plan which included inviting both sets of parents for a chat. Their main task was to give them information about Sophie and Donald's mental health, and to put their minds at rest by assuring them that the mental health condition of each was sufficiently stable to enable the couple to act as responsible adults. They also assured the parents that the nature of Sophie and Donald's relationship was such that they helped each other overcome mental health distress rather than hindered improvement – which the parents feared most. At the workers' suggestion, the couple and their parents then met socially on several occasions so that the parents got to know their child's choice of partner respectfully. Finally, the parents agreed to the marriage.

Who can act as an advocate?

This should be a voluntary worker who might be trained and supported by independently financed, paid staff, based outside the care agency. Or it could be the client's friend or a relative. In the absence of these, and when appropriate, you might as a paid worker be asked to act as an advocate – as in the previous case study.

ACTIVITY

Read the following case study, then answer the questions below.

Case study

Yvonne was a charming young woman, who had a habit of telling people things about herself which were not true. Those who knew her thought she did this in order to obtain attention.

One evening Yvonne fell asleep in her bedroom while watching TV, but soon woke up horrified to see Phillip, another client-resident, on top of her, tearing at her clothes with one hand and covering her mouth with the other. Having got what he came for, he left the room warning his victim that she had better keep quiet – because, he insisted, no one would believe her anyway.

Yvonne was distressed and it took her several days to pluck up the courage to tell her key worker Sarah about the incident. Sarah believed that this time Yvonne spoke the truth; yet, later, when speaking to her supervisor about it, Sarah began to doubt her first impression, thinking that her inexperience might make her a laughing stock in the eyes of her senior colleagues. Nevertheless, Phillip was interrogated, and convincingly denied Yvonne's allegations.

Yvonne thus continued to live in constant fear because she lived under the same roof as her attacker. Not surprisingly she confided in her mother when she came for her monthly visit. Outraged that the staff did not believe her, Yvonne's mother took her to see a solicitor to press charges against Phillip.

1 State which person or agency should provide advocacy support for Yvonne. Consider who would best be able to help Yvonne undertake the stressful task of seeing a solicitor and possibly going to court.

2 Ask your colleagues to join in a discussion regarding this case study. Is it good practice to give Yvonne an advocate chosen from among the carers of the residential setting on whose premises she experienced abuse? If not, explain why.

Citizen advocacy

This is when the client's concerns are taken up by an independent person. If advocacy is her main job and/or she is not a volunteer, her salary should come from independent sources – not from the health or local authorities. This is to guarantee commitment to the client's cause which can sometimes be impeded by conflicting interests. The case study above shows why this is so important.

In citizen advocacy, the advocate refers to her client as a partner, to indicate a relationship of equality and closeness of interests.

The advocate's role

The advocate's job is to represent a client's interests and wishes, in order to ensure that his health, social care and welfare needs and rights are understood, communicated and acted upon promptly by the relevant individuals and institutions.

Finding an advocate

In the previous case study, Yvonne's mother acted as her advocate initially, being the first person who wanted to make her daughter's voice heard. But you could argue that being her mother might lessen her objectivity. Besides, Yvonne needed professional support as well, so the care workers encouraged her to find an independent advocate outside the agency. They helped her get in touch with an advocacy worker in their locality. This was a volunteer, trained by and attached to a special agency, the Citizen's Advocacy Scheme for Mental Health, whose funds were independent. This was a far better option than to allow a worker from the residential setting itself, including Yvonne's key worker, to fill the advocate's role, because of the conflicting interests.

When conflicting interests arise

This can happen when a client seeks help from within the care setting for an adverse incident or abuse of her rights that happened there. The staff in the previous case study, for example, would find it difficult to protect one resident while causing stress to another, however objective they tried to be. A further source of bias might come from a desire to remain loyal to one's agency – for example to prevent any adverse publicity – which is a natural response. This is why it is important to give the client an independent advocate.

How advocacy helped Yvonne

Yvonne met Stuart who became her advocate, not only for that incident but on a long-term basis as well. When asked later about her experience, Yvonne claimed that she could never have got out of that impossible and terrifying situation without him. With Stuart's emotional support and his communication (which included his mediation) with other professionals, Yvonne eventually dropped the charges against Phillip. She also got an apology from the staff for not taking her complaint seriously. On her wishes she moved into a new home – a hostel for women only – where she felt secure and where she received counselling. None of this would have happened if her mother had not provided advocacy in the first instance, and if Yvonne had not been given an independent advocate.

Self-advocacy

Self-advocacy is a process by which the client has an opportunity to:

- communicate her wishes to the carer or other professionals;
- make informed choices regarding her care;
- defend her rights according to legislation and policies;
- seek and obtain information regarding her care, including obtaining access to personal files;
- make complaints following complaints procedures;
- receive support from people in a similar position by becoming a member of a self-advocacy group in her locality.

ACTIVITY

1 Find out from your supervisor about your agency's policies on advocacy and about your role in them. In what situations will you be expected to represent the client's interests, and to whom?

2 Find out about the advocacy network (or similar resources) in your area. Get in touch with them to find out how they operate.

3 If your agency employs advocates from outside, find out about its policies on confidential personal information. How much, for example, will an advocate need to be told about the client?

ACTIVITY

1 Ask a colleague to play the role of a professional while you take on the role of a client. Try to enact a situation within a care network in which you have been wronged in some way. For example:

- not given a choice of where to live;
- made to undergo treatment you did not approve of, although you were not sectioned (see Mental Health Act, section 1.5);
- not given a chance to give your views on a matter concerning you;
- not given your welfare entitlements.

2 You are the wronged client and you wish to be your own advocate. What do you say to the professional in question? Say it to your colleague. What do you wish to do? For example, do you wish to pursue your complaint further or are you satisfied with the explanation which you are given?

3 How do you evaluate the effectiveness of your speaking or acting for yourself?

4 Change the roles and consider another example. Discuss the outcomes. Seek the opportunity to share your experiences with your care team.

Self-advocacy groups

Client-led groups are rapidly growing in numbers, which shows that clients have the desire and the motivation to communicate with and educate carers about their needs. The range of interests and issues which these groups serve is very wide. For example, they may be campaigning against the use of ECT (see section 1.2) and compulsory medication, or mainly concerned with self-support.

Service users' meetings

These might have different names, usually chosen by the clients, for example House User Group, Patients' Council, or Residents' Association. The meetings are held by the clients in order to discuss issues such as:

- how to help themselves gain more control over their lives and their mental health services;
- educating workers about the involvement of the clients as the service users;
- contributing to the recruitment of new staff members;
- how to influence planning and management of mental health services;
- campaigning for particular issues concerning individual clients or the whole group.

If the clients choose, a staff representative may also be present. Representatives from the user groups are often sent to meetings of professionals to communicate the clients' wishes and take part in decision making.

Major problems with self-advocacy and client empowerment

Professionals are the major obstacle to clients gaining control over their care and their lives, often through their paternal attitude towards clients whom

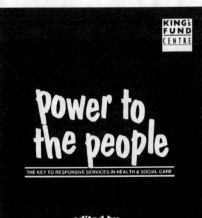

KING'S FUND CENTRE

power to the people

THE KEY TO RESPONSIVE SERVICES IN HEALTH & SOCIAL CARE

edited by
Liz Winn

they see as helpless. In addition, the willingness to share power, such as that derived from making decisions about care, is a challenge for workers which will not go away. This is borne out by the growing strength and achievements of service user groups, despite the poor funding for their work.

This is why your first step in changing the power balance may include changing your own views and attitudes towards clients with mental health problems. Treating them with dignity and respect at all times is a good start.

ACTIVITY

1 Find out about clients' meetings in you care setting:

- How frequently do they occur?
- How many clients are likely to attend?
- Who chairs the meetings?
- How are decisions made?
- How are clients' views, suggestions and decisions communicated to staff?

2 If such meetings do not take place in your care setting, find out why. Then get in touch with another agency in your area where such meetings are held. After speaking to staff and clients of that agency, put down your reasons for encouraging clients' meetings in your care setting. Then give them to your supervisor.

Self-advocacy packs

Some self-advocacy groups produce packs which provide information for clients on how to act and speak for themselves.

Crisis cards

These are carried by clients who want a named person of their choice to be contacted in the event of a mental health crisis – for example, before sectioning (see section 1.5). The nominee, that is the individual whose name is on this card, could be anyone: a professional, a friend or a relative.

CRISIS CARD
Advocacy South-East

Name of the cardholder: ....

Address: ....

....

Important: If anyone finds me, the cardholder, in a state which suggests that I am experiencing mental health distress or crisis as a result of which I appear unable or unwilling to co-operate in decisions regarding the best course of action to be taken, please contact the person named overleaf who has agreed to act on my behalf as my advocate.

Name and address of my advocate:

....

....

Telephone number:

Home: .... Work: ....

Other important information:

Signed: Date: ....

Front and back of a crisis card from a fictional self-advocacy organisation

---

ACTIVITY

1 Find out about crisis cards in your locality. Ask your local self-advocacy organisation to send you samples.

2 With your supervisor's permission, talk to clients to find out their views about the desirability and effectiveness of crisis cards.

<table>
<tr></tr>
</table>

ACTIVITY

1 Write to at least one of the organisations listed opposite and obtain information about their work and publications. For example, Survivors Speak Out can supply books and papers on topical and controversial issues in mental health and treatment, some written by clients; they also need 'allies' – professionals who support their work.

2 Obtain information from any of these organisations about self-advocacy groups in your area. Ask them to send you an information sheet, poster or leaflet which you could place on a notice board in your care setting for the clients to see.

Examples of mental health service user (self-advocacy) groups

Mindlink
c/o MIND
15–19 The Broadway
London E15 4BQ
Tel. 0181 519 2122

Survivors Speak Out (SSO)
34 Osnaburgh Street
London NW1 3ND
Tel. 0171 916 5472

UK Advocacy Network (UKAN)
Suite 302
Premier House
14 Cross Burgess Street
Sheffield S1 2HG
Tel. 0114 275 3131 (ext. 325) or 0114 272 8171

Further reading

★ *Guidelines on Advocacy for Mental Health Workers* by Jim Read and Jan Wallcraft, published by MIND Publications in 1994, is a positive pro-advocacy publication obtainable from MIND.

3.9 Monitoring and reviewing work with clients

Individual work with clients (as well as group work) usually needs to proceed through five stages: assessing, planning, monitoring, reviewing and ending.

Stage 1 Assessing Assessing client's needs, needs of carer and available resources.

Stage 2 Planning Planning time (carer's, client's and other professionals') and resources (material, skills and money); setting up goals.

Stage 3 Monitoring Record keeping; overviewing the helping process; directing helping towards set goals; examining the relevance of goals.

Stage 4 Reviewing Reviewing goals with client, supervisor and other carers.

Stage 5 Ending Agreeing to end with client and supervisor; summarising work with client and saying goodbye; writing up ending summary; closing or transferring files; communicating outcomes to all involved in client's care.

The process of working

The content of each of the five stages described does not have to follow the same rigid pattern on all occasions. For instance, if your task demands that you see a client only once or twice, the stages of working might be fewer and simpler. No matter what you are given to do, you will always have to do some assessment and planning (Stages 1 and 2), even if it is just thinking the task through and rehearsing in your head how you will proceed.

As you proceed with the work itself, you will have to keep an eye on how things are going (Stages 3 and 4), while your record keeping and other administrative tasks will have to comply with the practice of your agency (Stage 5).

ACTIVITY

1 Choose two clients with whom you have finished working. If this is not possible, choose clients with whom you are currently working. Then, bearing in mind the five stages described earlier, write down precisely what you did or intend to do at each stage. Be as concrete as possible. For example, you might write:

> Stage 1: I shall see Mary Rilke on 4 December at 10.30 a.m. to assess her need for an application for funds to

buy furniture for her new flat. I prepared myself by finding out about where we can apply for money and I got the necessary forms.

2 If you finished working with these clients and did not do all the five stages described earlier, can you see, in retrospect, whether it would have made any difference if you had included all five stages? If so, what?

Reviewing

Each care setting has its own guidelines and practices on how and when to review the care plans of individual clients. Usually this is done by holding meetings with the professionals involved in the client's care when some important decision has to be made, such as whether to move a client to a new environment. The client should always be present for at least part of the review meeting. Sometimes a review of individual tasks might be carried out as part of a larger care programme. For example, your supervisor might suggest that you meet with your client to discuss her progress regarding her participation in the cookery group.

You and the client

Involving the client at the different stages of caring fosters independence. Remember, clients are individuals, and the best way of learning about what works for each one is to ask him or her directly. Encourage clients to tell you what they find helpful and what they do not. To do this effectively, you should be prepared to receive constructive criticism as well as praise. Examples of questions you could ask are given below.

Examples of questions for reviewing
- How do you feel about what we have done so far (or what we did last week, or during our last meeting)?
- What did you find most helpful?
- What did you find least helpful?
- What (or which part of the task) did you find most difficult and why?
- How do you think we can improve our way of dealing with this problem? (State the problem.)

- What are your thoughts on that particular kind of help? (State the specific help which you have given or have provided for the client.)
- What ideas or suggestions do you have as to what we should do?
- What would you like me to do differently?
- What do you think we should do now – for example, finish our work by a certain date in the near future, do something else, do more of the same, or do the difficult part of the task again?

Defensiveness

Try to avoid being defensive – justifying yourself, using lengthy explanations which have no direct relevance to the criticism made, or getting angry and attacking the client by criticising him when he tells you something you do not want to hear about your work or conduct. It is natural to want to protect yourself from other people's unpleasant opinions to maintain your self-esteem. It should help you to receive criticism if you remember that it is not you as a person that is being criticised, but only one aspect of what you do – which you can change. By not accepting criticism, you will never learn or develop as a care worker and as a person.

Dealing with criticism

If you get angry or upset, count to ten inwardly to prevent yourself from acting without thinking. It is unprofessional to show anger and defensiveness towards clients. Instead, stop and try to think of a constructive response. If none comes to you, you could, for example, say that you will think about it. Always thank the client for any feedback.

Reviewing your use of time

Time is one of the most valuable commodities, not least because mental health services are commonly underfunded so that care agencies often have to function with insufficient workers.

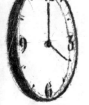

Time is precious: use it carefully

ACTIVITY

1 Think about how you spend your time at work. Do you have such a thing as a typical week at work? If so, note down how much time you spend on:

- practical tasks for or with clients;
- emotional support or befriending;
- group activities with clients, including outings;
- meetings with colleagues and other professionals;
- supervision;
- administration, such as record keeping and letter writing;

- in-service training – attendance on courses or staff discussions;
- chatting with colleagues or clients, not as a part of your work but as social interaction;
- other (specify).

2 Looking at your time chart, indicate where you should allow more time (e.g. helping clients with practical tasks) and where less (e.g. administration). Discuss your findings with your supervisor to explore ways of improving your use of time.

4 Working with people in groups

4.1 Functions of groups

People have always formed themselves into groups to ensure the survival of individual members and the species as a whole. There are certain fundamental functions which all groups aim to fulfil, be it a tribe in West Africa, an organisation in the UK such as one providing employment to its members, a communal group such as a kibbutz in Israel, or the members of a nuclear family.

ACTIVITY

1 List ways in which you think you benefit from being part of a family or part of a group such as a circle of friends, colleagues or a community.

2 Ask a friend or co-worker to share with you some thoughts on how being a member of various groups is beneficial for him or her.

Most of us would agree that being part of a group gives:

- a sense of belonging;
- a feeling of togetherness and safety;
- the companionship of people similar to ourselves;
- an opportunity for social interaction and self-expression;
- support and help when we need it.

Groups as a means of social support

Many people who experience mental health distress lack social support. This can be for a variety of reasons. Some live far away from their families or have broken contact with them; others do not have anyone close who can give them support when they need it. In some cases, when an individual's behaviour is driven by extreme and often unpredictable changes in mood, deep depression or delusions (see section 1.2), those close to him or her may find it very difficult to cope. Their inability to deal with the situation may lead them to distance themselves from the emotionally troubled individual, who experiences this as rejection. The vicious circle then continues as the person experiencing mental health problems is likely to shy away from people even more for fear of rejection.

This is why both formal and informal group activities are so important in mental health care; they are therapeutic and can compensate for inadequate social support from the family or society at large.

ACTIVITY

Read the following case study, then list at least three ways in which the client benefits from being an active member of the group.

Case study

Maureen is in her 60s and has a 30-year history of mental health difficulties. She attends a 'communication through writing and art' group. At one meeting she is asked to read her work aloud – a single verse of a poem. There are about 11 other clients and a care worker, all sitting in a circle, attentive. They listen as she reads:

Have physical illness
you get fruit, flowers and smiles
have mental illness
people run from you for miles.

One by one, the group members begin to give comments on how they understand and experience the verse. They share their own views and feelings about the subject expressed, which is very close to their hearts. Someone comments on how well Maureen has put her views and feelings into words.

The benefits of attending a group

The above case study demonstrates the benefits of attending a group. Firstly Maureen has an opportunity to express herself in the presence of a group of people on a subject which represents the reality of her experiences. She is expressing herself in an atmosphere where she knows she will be understood. By sharing her thoughts and feelings on such a sensitive issue with others, Maureen makes positive steps towards starting new friendships or cementing old ones.

Secondly, by reading out her poem on this painful topic, she receives sympathy and fellow-feeling from other participants, which will show her that she is not alone in experiencing rejection and isolation due to mental health distress.

Thirdly, someone comments about her skill at writing, which will be beneficial for Maureen's sense of worth, contributing to her developing a better opinion of herself.

From this example you can see how active participation in a group activity can help the client:

- express thoughts and feelings;
- feel accepted by others;
- develop a better sense of worth;
- make new friends.

ACTIVITY

Make a list of the positive features that you gain from your own activities, at work and on your course, excluding the financial gain or acquisition of a certificate.

A sense of identity

As human beings we have an ability to form our identity, an idea of ourselves as individuals. Then we form our personal opinions and feelings towards that identity, attaching to it certain values. This is what we mean by the term *self-esteem*. Both processes – defining ourselves (formation of identity) and developing self-esteem (values attached to that identity) – involve some kind of comparison or 'measuring' of ourselves against others. This means that others are necessary for us in order to develop and maintain our identity as human beings.

Identity and groups

In one of the Radio 4 programmes in the series *All in the Mind*, psychiatrist Anthony Clare talks about the 'bonding' (feeling of togetherness and emotional attachment) which exists in groups regardless of their nature. In trying to explain the popularity of groups, Professor Clare points out that our first learning about ourselves takes place within a group, that is within a family or its substitute. He states that 'before we know who we are as individuals, we have to know who we are as a group'.

Self-esteem and mental health

Self-esteem is a part of our identity. Emotionally damaged people are likely to have a low self-esteem. This means that they do not value themselves much as individuals and their identity needs to be redefined so that they may form a more positive opinion of themselves. Being part of a group with which they find something in common can help this process of healing, through the feedback which they will receive from others and through comparison and identification with individual group members.

A need for activity

Besides the social and psychological benefits to clients, group activity can help to fill in the long periods of unemployment and inactivity which are a frequent consequence of mental health distress.

ACTIVITY

Read the following case study, then list at least six ways in which you believe John and Peter will benefit from the cookery group.

Case study

John moved into a residential home a couple of months ago. Previous to this he was hospitalised for six months due to a 'breakdown' after he lost his job as a chef in a small hotel. John used to enjoy cooking very much, but since his hospitalisation and transfer into the home, all his meals have been served to him. He liked that during the initial emotional crisis because he could not have coped with the responsibility of cooking for himself, but lately he has become restless with nothing to do. He has developed a habit of pacing up and down the lounge all day long, feeling useless and frustrated.

There are 12 residents, but the only person John seems to communicate with is Peter. Perhaps this is because Peter is well on the way to recovery, and there are rumours of his moving into his own flat in the near future. Unlike John, Peter never learned to cook even the simplest of meals. His sister, who had unexpectedly committed suicide, used to do everything for him. Peter is also restless having nothing to do, and the two men enrol for the cookery group at the first opportunity.

Using the above case study, it is evident that:

- the group will help structure John and Peter's time;
- it will take away some of the boredom;
- it will teach Peter some important skills necessary for independent living;
- it can help develop hidden talents and rediscover John's forgotten skills;
- it can provide a sense of self-respect and, in Peter's case, help improve the self-esteem associated with learning new skills;
- for John, who is relearning the skill, it can provide an opportunity to inspire and teach others;

- learning in groups can nurture a sense of responsibility and motivation, because the presence of others can inject enthusiasm to do well;
- new friendships may be formed which can then exist outside the group.

Promoting better health

Group activities, such as sports, walking and relaxation, promote better physical health. Sport can also have a therapeutic value when it is used to use up surplus energy and anger. Broadly speaking, any kind of group activity conducted with the carer's support and the clients' willing participation can be therapeutic.

4.2 Setting up groups

When setting up a formal group – as opposed to an informal one, such as taking clients out to see a film or concert – you need to consider several questions such as what kind of group activity to have, where it should take place, and who will attend it.

Where to have a group?

Where a group meets depends on facilities such as the space available and its accessibility, as well as on clients' needs.

Your own care setting is an obvious choice, but you may also have the option of running a group elsewhere, for example in a local church hall, psychiatric hospital or a hostel where more dependent people go to stay for a while when they are discharged from hospital. You may wish to share the running of a group with another professional, such as an occupational therapist or colleagues from an adjacent care centre, perhaps using that centre's facilities. The last example is particularly relevant if your aim is to liaise with clients in the locality so that they can get to know about your care setting and use it when the need arises.

Running a group in another care setting could be viewed as a form of outreach work, whose aim is to attract those who may in the near future benefit from what your care setting has to offer.

Groups in the community

These can make your clients feel that they are truly part of the community. An example would be a tea group run in a church hall, where clients can mix with others in the locality. Alternatively, you might wish to make a special arrangement with those in charge of community facilities to take your clients to a local sports centre for swimming or aerobics for example – activities which, due to lack of confidence, some clients might not do without a care worker.

Access to groups

Make sure that the venue you choose for your group is the best one available in regard to its accessibility. For instance, a room on the ground level will

> **ACTIVITY**
>
> With your supervisor and co-workers, explore the facilities and material available for groups in your care setting. What, if any, groups are presently running in your workplace? Try to identify a need for something different which can benefit your clients.

> **ACTIVITY**
>
> *1* Find out about groups running in other centres in the area where you work. Find out about available facilities, such as space for groups.
>
> *2* By speaking to professionals in other care settings for similar clients in your locality, explore the needs for a specific type of group activity. You could ring the centre and speak to someone in charge there or ask to speak to the worker who is experienced in running groups.

enable an older person who cannot climb stairs to attend. Provision of a crèche would enable single parents to attend, who can often be isolated.

Gathering information about your clients' needs and interests

Clients are individuals and so their interests will vary from local history and hiking, for example, to watching old films, drawing or just being with other people and exchanging views on current affairs, food or fashion.

Sometimes clients' interests will coincide with their care needs. For example, homemaking may well be a priority for a client who is waiting to move into his own home after several years spent in a residential care setting. However, at other times you may find that clients express interests based on unrealistic expectations. For example, a client might say he wants to learn how to run his own business when he is still, in fact, highly dependent on carers – unable to handle money, keep doctor's appointments or take care of his personal appearance.

As a carer, your role is to make your clients' care needs appear interesting so that they want to join in activities which will help them towards independent living. Your own enthusiasm, regardless of how mundane the activity seems, is important.

ACTIVITY

1 Talk to your clients and find out about the activities which interest them or which they used to enjoy when they were well.

- Are there skills which they feel they need to learn or relearn to help them towards independent living?
- Are there new skills they should develop in order to adapt to their new circumstances?

2 Write down each client's interests and needs. The needs may be of a practical nature, such as learning how to prepare a simple but nutritious meal, or they may require a social skill, such as how to communicate more effectively and with greater confidence. Or they may be of an emotional nature, such as finding a way of expressing one's emotions in socially acceptable ways (e.g. through painting, poetry or play reading). An example is provided opposite.

Clients' interests and needs

Name	Current activities	Needs and skills to learn	Interests and aspirations	Suggested groups to supply needs
Christine Taylor	Music group, Wed. 3–5 p.m.	Women's health information for over 50s	Teas and dancing; play reading and acting	Women's health information group; drama
Raymond Jones	Therapy group, Mon. 10–12 a.m. Learning keyboard (WP) skills Thurs. 2–4 p.m.	Communication and assertiveness; need to stop smoking	Writing poetry; discussion of current affairs	Anxiety management; assertiveness training
Bill Rodgers	None	Food preparation; finance management	Gardening; woodwork; swimming	Cookery group; independent living training

Be aware

Try to prompt gently and be persistent until you are sure you have explored your clients' interests and needs thoroughly. The lack of motivation of your clients, caused by their psychological state or by medication, may easily give you the impression that there is very little, if anything, they would like to do. Try to inject some positive self-image: encourage whenever you can.

Your attitude towards the group activity should be positive and enthusiastic. At the same time, be careful that you do not mishear your client in your enthusiasm to sign her up for a particular group – always respect her wishes.

Use your skills and interests

Your own interests, skills and potential are valuable in this work and you should by all means try to develop and utilise them as best you can; but remember that your clients' needs come first. If you can match your clients' needs with your own, think yourself lucky. If you cannot, flexibility and willingness to learn new skills and expand your own interests will be both necessary and rewarding.

What kind of group?

One way of dividing groups is according to their activities. Here are some examples:

- life skills, such as cooking, homemaking, finance management, health awareness and personal care;
- personal development and individual interest groups, such as painting, writing, photography and walking;
- social skills development groups which explore and develop assertiveness and communication skills;
- various types of 'therapy' groups – psychotherapy, occupational therapy, drama and dance (or movement) and art therapy;
- sports and leisure groups – swimming, running, chess, Scrabble, etc.

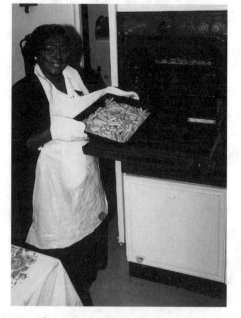

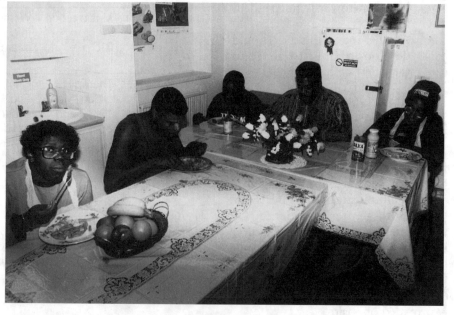

A cookery group
(a) The group leader

(b) The group eating what they have cooked

The functions of various groups should not be viewed rigidly, because many groups have more than one function.

The kind of group you choose to run will also depend on:

- the objectives you propose to achieve;
- other activities taking place in your care setting;
- your own interests, and those of your co-workers for joint work;
- the number of clients who could benefit from such a group;
- the facilities available in your care setting or in other places with potential for groups in the local community.

Who is the group for?

This question is closely bound up with the group's aims. If you are working in a residential care setting, you may wish to make the group available not only to the resident clients but also to people attending local day centres, or to clients who live alone in the community. Here your objectives might be to provide an opportunity for your residents to make friends with clients who live more independently. Such friendships would be particularly beneficial for residents who are soon to move out into the community.

> **TO THINK ABOUT**
>
> Considering that social stigma and public attitudes towards people with mental health problems are usually founded on ignorance, prejudice and fear, how do you think such attitudes might be influenced when people from the local community mix and interact with your clients in a joint group activity?

> **CASE STUDY**
>
> Jova Gruich is a volunteer, making teas and snacks in the mental health day centre where he has made many friends since his first visit two years ago. He remembers the time when he first saw the poster in a local library about a creative writing group; it said 'All welcome'. He also recalls his surprise when the care worker who interviewed him before he joined the group asked him about his experience of mental health. 'None' he replied, puzzled. 'Why? Is that going to be the subject of your writing workshops?'
>
> Being new to the area, Jova hadn't realised that the address on the poster referred to a mental health day centre. But he often acted on impulse, and since he enjoyed his chat with Anne Creasy – the prospective group leader – he decided to give it a try.
>
> He never regretted that day. Tom Chapman, one of the clients, and Jova became good friends almost from the first meeting of the group. They discovered while chatting during a tea break that they read the same authors and had seen the same plays. They exchanged books and pieces of writing which each had done on their own, always encouraging each other to write.
>
> Eventually, Jova became a volunteer at the centre, working alongside several client-volunteers in the drop-in café, where he gradually made more friends. Tom has been out many times with Jova and his friends. His self-esteem and communication, as well as writing skills, have improved greatly since this friendship. But that's not all. All Jova's friends were told many good things about 'the centre' and its members which, inevitably, influenced their views about people with mental distress.

Including the community

You may decide (with your supervisor's approval) to allow people in the community to join your group, provided you have the space and your clients feel comfortable with this. Several local residents may wish to attend your group – as they might attend a course run by a local Adult Education Centre. This could be of tremendous value to your clients, who are bound to feel the social stigma associated with mental health problems. Having so-called 'normal' people attend the same group will go a long way to making your clients feel accepted. It might also provide a stepping stone for the more independent clients to gain confidence and enrol on a course in the local Adult Education Centre, and, by doing so, to truly integrate into the community.

4.3 Planning groups

In planning a group, you should first consider your objectives and aims. Objectives are goals, long-term targets which you believe the group can achieve; aims are ways in which you intend to achieve these goals. The easy way to remember this is to think of objectives by asking yourself *what* you want to achieve, and of aims by making it clear *how* you are going to do it.

Example of objectives
The objectives of a discussion group might be to provide clients with an opportunity to:

* express views and feelings on topical subjects;
* interact socially within a 'safe' supervised environment, encouraged, supported and guided by the care worker;
* make friends who have similar views;
* learn how to listen to others, even when their views are different.

Group objectives

Below are examples of objectives or goals for groups within mental health, the appropriateness of which will depend on the actual group activity.

* Help clients towards independent living.
* Help self-expression and communication.
* Develop and nurture social interaction so that clients may be aided in making new and maintaining old relationships.
* Facilitate learning of a particular skill needed for rehabilitation.
* Help clients structure time and relearn a sense of responsibility – for example, punctuality for meetings and preparation.

ACTIVITY

1 Decide what kind of group you wish to set up and, if possible, where it will take place.

2 Think of particular clients who will be involved. Now list in detail what your clients will gain from participating in your group.

TO THINK ABOUT

Having read the list of objectives for a discussion group given in the previous example, consider *how* you will achieve them (your aims).

ACTIVITY

1 Thinking about your particular care setting and the clients within it, describe a group activity which could fulfil the objective of helping the clients towards independent living.

2 List individual clients who might benefit from joining such a group.

3 Talk to these clients and find out how they feel about attending such a group.

Planning

Once you know your objectives and what kind of group you are going to run and where, you need to ask these questions:

- Will I run the group alone or with a co-worker?
- When shall I start the group?
- Who should attend? Who will?
- What should be the minimum and maximum numbers of participants?
- How many meetings or sessions will the group have?
- How long will each session be? Will there be a break in the middle?
- How will I recruit group members?
- Who will interview and admit clients into the group?

Talk to your supervisor

Your final decision about the details of running a group should always come after talking to your supervisor and getting her approval. There are several reasons for this, including the fact that any new project will have to fit in with other demands and activities which are already taking place or being planned.

How to recruit for groups

Several activities in this chapter involved talking to clients and colleagues in your care setting to find out what kind of group activity might be desirable and appropriate. But imagine that, besides your clients, you wish to make the group open to other people with mental health problems in your locality – to clients who, at the moment, do not use or even know about your care setting.

You could try to attract such people by putting a poster or notice in a public place such as a local library. Leave plenty of time before the group starts, so that potential participants can see the notice and plan their time to attend.

Creating a poster or a group information sheet

You do not have to be an artist to create a poster, but you must include essential information such as the starting date, location and contact number. You should also say if an interview is needed, to avoid disappointing people who might otherwise just turn up when the group is about to start.

Referrals from other professionals

If you wish other care professionals in your locality to refer their clients to your group, you will have to inform them about it well before it is due to start. Check with your supervisor about the policy of your care setting.

Confidentiality of received information

If other professionals (e.g. doctors, social workers, psychiatrists and psychiatric nurses) refer their clients to your group, they are likely to disclose confidential information to you – especially if you are responsible for interviewing to admit group members. Make sure that you treat such information with the utmost confidentiality and respect, and store it safely.

ACTIVITY

Find out about other groups in your care setting, or about groups which have been successful in the past. Then approach the colleagues responsible for running them and enquire how they went about recruiting clients.

By talking to your colleagues who have run groups you can benefit from their experience and, at the same time, not feel completely alone in your efforts to start a group.

ACTIVITY

Imagine that you have all the information you need about a group you are going to start in the near future, including the name of the group and when it will start. Create a poster which will be used to publicise your group. An example is given on page 108.

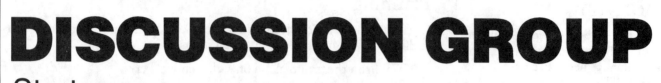

DISCUSSION GROUP

Starts on
Thursday 3rd September
3.00–5.00 p.m.

at

**St Mary's Lodge
(Ground Floor)
55 Albany Avenue
Newtown**

'It's good to talk ...'

ALL WELCOME

*For more information
            and
                an informal interview*

ring DAVE LEVI on 399 247

A poster for a discussion group

4.4 Group leadership

You might be entrusted to lead a group on your own, with the support and guidance of your supervisor. On the other hand, you might lead a group with a senior colleague or even a worker from another care setting. If you are going to lead a group with someone else, it is important to meet the colleague to agree on the role and tasks which each of you will have for each session.

Another option, if you and your colleagues are overworked and have no time for a full commitment to the group, is for two or more workers to take the group alternately. This is suitable for some types of groups such as swimming and baking, but is not recommended for groups where clients are likely to share personal information and express their feelings, such as in a creative writing or art group. This is because they need to build trust in a group leader and new faces may make them feel unsafe and vulnerable.

ACTIVITY

1 Think about your own experiences of being part of a group which had a leader or a tutor. Write a paragraph describing how the tutor led the group.

2 List what you liked about this kind of leadership, giving your reasons.

3 List what you did not like about it and why.

4 If you do not have any group experience yourself, think of a group you would like to join. Note down your expectations of its leader.

Qualities of a group leader

The previous activity may have produced some answers related to the personal qualities of a group leader, tutor or teacher from your own experience. The person who left you with a memory of a positive group experience is likely to have had some or all of the qualities described below.

Positive attitude

The group leader should have a positive and enthusiastic attitude towards the group activities, as well as towards the group members. A half-hearted or reluctant way of relating to the group will not produce a stimulating, motivating atmosphere for your clients.

Patience

Allowing each individual to communicate or to complete an activity in his own time (within the time structured for the group) and in his individual way is important for the client's self-esteem. It may also be important if he is learning a life skill. Remember, just because someone takes a long time to peel and dice an apple, this does not mean he will not learn how to bake an excellent apple pie.

Encouragement

Every group leader should develop the ability to encourage all group members to participate in the group's activities. Also, because group activities have a social dimension – that is, they include social interaction between participants such as sharing ideas and feelings – the group leader should encourage all members to take an active part in the social aspects of the group.

Awareness

Awareness is seeing, hearing, noticing and being fully conscious of what is going on around you. Self-awareness is your knowledge and appreciation of what is going on inside you: your thoughts, feelings, reactions to others, and your own behaviour. Although both types of awareness are important when you are a group leader, awareness of others is crucial. This means that at all times during the group's activities you should observe your clients, their interaction with yourself and others (or lack of it), and their activities.

Only by being aware of what is going on will you be able to encourage, instruct and guide, or defuse the situation when misunderstanding, conflict or problems occur (see also section 2.5).

The role of the group leader

The role of the group leader – which is the facilitation of a group – may vary from group to group and from setting to setting. Nevertheless, there are certain tasks which each worker is expected to fulfil when starting a group.

- Prepare materials which you need for each session well in advance; also plan an outline for each meeting so that you give it a structure within which the group's activities can take place.
- If the group members include people from outside your care setting, you should introduce yourself at the beginning of the first meeting.
- Make sure the members know important details about the group such as its aims, planned activities, duration, breaks (if any), refreshments and other practical arrangements.
- If participants do not know each other you should help them to introduce themselves, whenever possible in their own words.
- Get the participants to help generate ideas for sessions and prepare for meetings by, for example, bringing materials or items for the group (if applicable).
- Make sure that you always begin the group at the planned time, remembering that you are setting an example for others.
- Make sure that all participants are informed of cancellations or rescheduling of a session as soon as possible.
- Create order and discipline. Although it is important to create a relaxed atmosphere and give encouragement, you also need to convey to clients that certain kinds of behaviour are acceptable, while others are not. Explain that this is for the benefit of all participants and to help the group achieve its objectives.

There will undoubtedly be other tasks which you will be expected to do as a group leader. For example, you are likely to be responsible for the finances of the group: keeping receipts for the purchase of materials or other expenses such as the group's outings.

Keeping written records

The main reasons for keeping written records for groups are that:

1   they help you monitor the progress of the group;

ACTIVITY

Give at least two good reasons why keeping written records of your group's meetings is a valuable practice.

2 they help you monitor the involvement of individual participants in the group's activities, and their social interaction both with each other and with yourself;

3 they give useful statistics for your care setting, which can help in evaluating its work;

4 if you are working towards an NVQ or SVQ, they can provide evidence of your skill.

Creating a recording sheet

Your care setting may already have forms for recording group sessions. If not, create your own and make copies for future use. Here is an example of a recording sheet to help you get started.

Recording sheet for the play-reading group

Run by: Ann Miller

Session No. 3   *Date*: 12.5.199X

Numbers of attenders: 5

Present: Ben Thompson, Audrey Brown, Mary Francis, Bob Winters, Winifred Bell

Comments on the members' activities: Mary Francis was 20 minutes late due to having to go to get her injection. All members read their parts willingly and several of them brought items of clothing to make their parts more realistic.

Comments on the members' interaction: Benjamin Thompson was the only member who did not join in the laughter caused by other members trying to act as they read their parts.

    Audrey was more social than usual – helping others to find their place in the book when their turn came.

Signed *A. Miller* (group leader)

You can include other subheadings relating to specific information you want to find out. For example, you could keep a track of the numbers of men and women attenders if you suspect gender imbalance.

Checklist

If you have followed the section on groups so far and taken part in the activities, you should by now have the knowledge to answer the following questions:

1 What kind of group activity do you want to set up?
2 Where will the group meet or go?
3 Who will attend the group?
4 What are its objectives?
5 How can your group fulfil the individual needs of your clients?
6 What qualities do you need to develop to be a good group leader?
7 How will you recruit participants?
8 What are your duties as a group leader?

ACTIVITY

1 Arrange to attend a group meeting in your care setting. Always check first with your supervisor. Observe the group activity and write down what you see, paying attention to points such as:

- self-expression of participants, through communication as well as through the activity;
- interaction between clients;
- interaction with the group leader;

2 How successful is the group socially? Is there a balanced social interaction or are one or two clients taking up most of the time and so getting most attention from the group leader and others present?

3 How is the leader facilitating the group? Would you do something differently? What and why?

4.5 The group process

An informal group, such as a Christmas party at the centre or sitting with clients in a cinema, might not require the same kind of intense concentration and alertness from a care worker as a formal group. This is because informal groups usually have an external focus – music, games, food and drink, or a film for clients to watch. This does not mean that you should close your eyes to listen to the music during a party at the centre, for example, and forget your most important responsibility – the clients' safety. However, in a formal group where clients have hardly anything to focus on apart from the group's activity, which is facilitated by you, you might feel that your job is more demanding.

Group norms

Groups have norms – a set of minimum values and behaviours which members are expected to follow. Many groups have norms which are implicit rather than explicit, usually defined by the context. For example, a group of patients sitting in a GP's waiting room know what is expected of them; the context of waiting in a surgery for your turn clearly defines how each member behaves. If a couple, for example, walked in with a loud tape-recorder, performed a tap dance, and passed around a purse for collection, patients and staff would probably find such behaviour distasteful. Yet, if this couple did their dance in a high street crowded with Christmas shoppers, the same people would be likely to stop to watch and reward the dancers with spare change.

In these examples it is the context where the dance is performed which has changed. A doctor's surgery has an implicit rule of order, of subdued conversation or silence. A high street, on the other hand, suggests a greater range of behaviour, especially at certain times of the year and on special occasions.

Boundaries

Boundaries are limits of accepted behaviours; we are all ruled by limits, although they will vary depending on the situation. It is often necessary to set boundaries in order to ensure the smooth running of a centre. Above all, clients with a history of emotional difficulties need certain limits of behaviour which will teach them, by example within a care setting, about the world at large.

Testing the limits of boundaries

Some people with emotional difficulties and great emotional needs have difficulty in accepting limits, either because they have not learned to when growing up, or because their need to make up for the attention, love and acceptance they never had is so great that they will try to 'test' the worker – not unlike a child who tests how far he can misbehave with a parent or new teacher. Of course, there are other reasons for breaking boundaries. For example, someone who always acts on impulse to satisfy his own desire might never have learned how to postpone his gratification or have more consideration for others.

Some explicit rules may be necessary

Some groups need to have more explicitly defined rules or boundaries to create a safe environment and the order necessary for achieving the group's objectives.

Examples of boundaries

The boundaries set will depend very much on the group's activity, although some boundaries might apply to many groups. For example, if the group's activity demands concentration, such as during a creative writing or art group, all participants should agree to remain quiet during these periods. Another example might be agreement about when to have a tea break and for how long.

Ground rules

Establishing a set of ground rules for the group can go a long way to clarifying expectations, helping individuals to learn boundaries and the group to develop its norms. You may at first think that having rules sounds too

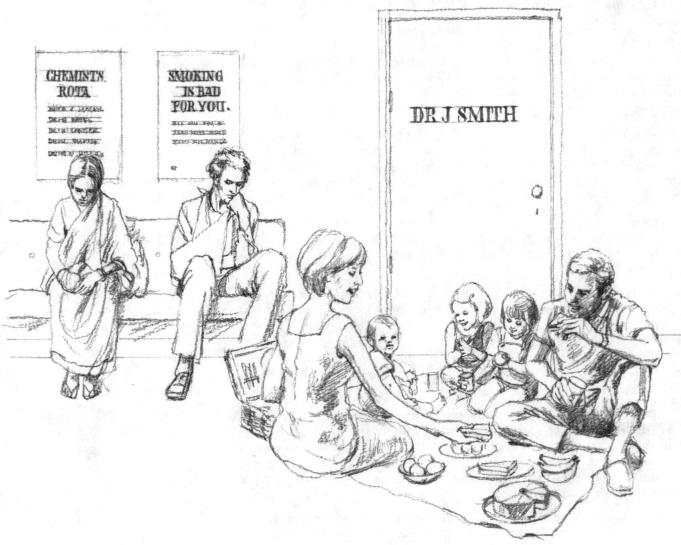

Boundaries have broken down here

authoritarian. However, the opposite may be true. Provided you take care in how you introduce such rules to the group members and how you deal with situations when the rules are broken, ground rules are a support not a restraint.

Striving for balance

You may rightly want to avoid making too many rules for your clients, not least because the process will make them feel institutionalised, while spontaneity of self-expression will suffer. But be careful that, in striving to avoid making rules, you do not leave clients confused and apprehensive due to lack of guidance.

Establishing boundaries in a creative way

1 Decide in advance (before you meet with the group members) which aspects of the clients' behaviour are important for the group's activity to be performed successfully. Make notes of these so that you can refer to them later, especially during the first meeting with the group members. For example, you might decide that observation of silence and remaining seated during the group's activity are very important, that the members should abstain from eating or drinking during the group's activity period, and so on.

2 Take a large piece of paper and a thick felt pen to the first meeting of your group. After the members' introductions, sum up the aims of the group and justify a need for certain ground rules by referring to the aims. Then ask participants to contribute in creating the group's ground rules, getting one of the clients to write them down.

3 Listen to your clients' suggestions and write them down legibly. If the ideas are not expressed clearly, help the clients by gentle probing and encouragement, summing up their points succinctly. If you do this, your clients will feel that you respect their opinions. They will also feel that they made the rules, rather than you, the worker, who represents authority. Remember, many people take pleasure in being rebellious against authority.

4 Prompt your clients until all the points you wrote down before the session are covered. You will be surprised how well your clients can work together to create the group's norms. If something important has been omitted, ask open questions such as:

- What do you think should be the limit on being late? (You may wish to make suggestions, such as no limit, up to 15 minutes, up to 30 minutes.)
- How should we deal with persistent latecomers? (Again, give suggestions if appropriate.)
- How do you think the group should react if someone is repeatedly disruptive?

5 Agree to bring the list of ground rules to every meeting, explaining that this will be a reminder to the group of the commitment they have made. It will also inform those who join the group later about what is expected of them, so that they can easily discover some of the group's norms. Another reason for having the list at all times is so it can be reviewed, modified or extended, if necessary, as the group progresses.

Do not underestimate the power of group pressure. You do not need to be a loud, strict disciplinarian; rather, get your clients to discipline for you.

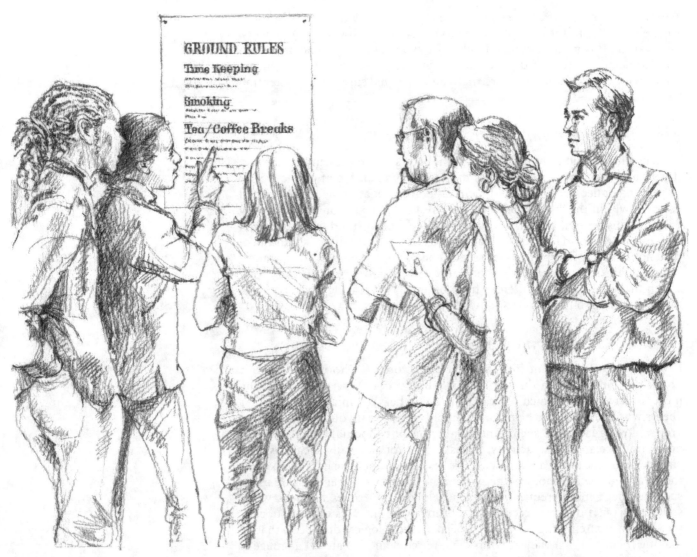

GROUND RULES

Time Keeping

Smoking

Tea / Coffee Breaks

Group ground rules

Group dynamics

Every group has its own dynamics – the changing nature of interaction and relationships between members. Once a group has started to meet, its dynamics can be observed on two levels, usually happening at the same time. The *task level* reflects whatever the group has set out to do; the *social level* reflects its social interaction. Your role as group leader is to monitor this process on both levels so that you can facilitate it. This means you need to be aware of the following:

- What are the individual group members doing? For example, if they have to use equipment, are they handling it safely? Are they carrying out the agreed activity or doing something else, perhaps because they have not understood your instructions?
- How do the group members interact with each other? For instance, is there a conflict between any of them? Who is taking the role of leader and who is demanding too much attention from others or yourself?

Give support to all individuals

We all have preferences concerning people we like, dislike and towards whom we are indifferent. It is natural for you to feel similarly towards your clients. Be aware of this natural human tendency in yourself; only by acknowledging and being aware of it do you stand a chance of consciously influencing your own behaviour, making sure that you give equal support and attention to all.

Members who stand out from others

A client who is noticeably different from the others who represent the majority (for example, one who is physically disabled, from a different ethnic origin, or gay) might need your sensitivity and support in her attempt to be accepted as equal within the group. This does not mean that you should deliberately focus on this person; by doing so you would make her stand out even more, which is likely to make her feel uncomfortable. So, while you should take care not to make it appear a big issue if one of your clients is, for instance, blind or Chinese, you should also not ignore it, especially when a characteristic which makes the person different from others has a bearing upon how she fits within the group's norms and how she participates in its activities.

Include clients from other cultures

If your group has a client from another ethnic origin, who is not fluent in English or familiar with the mainstream cultural norms, try to find out the most effective way in which you can help him or her. You might involve other clients who are willing to help. For example, be aware if you or other clients are employing language such as regional terms or colloquial expressions, or even jargon related to an activity. If this is how you normally speak, ask the client whether he has heard such expressions before, and if he has not, explain the meaning. Notice, too, whether you or the other group members are using such language more frequently than usual; this sometimes happens when someone from a different race or subculture is present. It is often a subconscious way of attempting to keep people at a psychological distance – that is, making them feel that they are outsiders, rejected and isolated. Language is a powerful weapon, but it can also build bridges between the known and unknown, the familiar and strange, and in so doing replace fear by freedom and hatred by love. Make sure that you use language in a positive way.

Value differences

Differences among your clients can bring richness and liveliness to groups, as well as the opportunity to question and challenge some stereotypical assumptions based on lack of knowledge and direct experience. As a group leader, and also as a care worker, it is your job to try to convey to others the value of individual differences. Human diversity is a natural and positive thing, reflecting the richness and complexity of human nature. If you treat everyone with respect, sensitivity and tolerance, your clients will soon follow your example.

Pay attention to clients with physical limitations

Always check with your supervisor before you consider recruiting individuals with more severe forms of physical disability for a group which will consist mainly of the physically able. For example, you must recognise that taking a client who has lost a limb on an outing will cause problems if it includes energetic uphill walking and uneven terrain.

When problems arise

Sometimes people with mental health difficulties behave unpredictably: a client may suddenly over-react to something another client has said or done, or she may become extremely distressed in a particular situation outside the care setting. She may become unco-operative or try to prevent other group members from carrying on with the group's activities. You have to be resourceful in dealing with problems that arise during a group activity; this comes with experience. Getting to know the clients well will help you notice early signs of agitation and take steps to avoid problems.

ACTIVITY

1 List the worst problems which you imagine, realistically, can happen within a group meeting of people with mental health distress:

- in a care setting;
- in a public place, during an outing.

2 Having made such a list, ask your supervisor to explain the policy of your care setting in regard to these events.

Prevent problems by careful selection

You may never be able to avoid all problems, but you can strive to minimise them. By carefully selecting the people who join your group, you may prevent incidents which would be damaging to your clients and spoil the enjoyment of the group's members. This may not be an easy task when you are interviewing people who are less well known to you, such as clients from another care setting. Read their case notes and find out from the professionals to whom they are known about their group attendance in the past and their general behaviour. If you do this, you will soon discover if a client is known to be disruptive or abusive to others, or if a client's mental distress is of such a nature that the group's activity may cause her even more distress.

Saying 'no' is a part of caring

Your aim is not to be punitive towards someone who might be causing problems because of her unbalanced emotional state; rather, it is to protect such a client from embarrassment and the adverse reactions which her behaviour might trigger in others, as well as to protect other clients. As pointed out in the section on boundaries, some clients may need strict rules set out for them; this is all part of their rehabilitation. Saying 'no' to clients is part of caring for them.

Ending the group

This is an important part of any formal group activity which involves a number of meetings of participants over a period.

TO THINK ABOUT

What feelings do you think would affect your clients on the last session of a group of people who have met regularly for four months?

Ending may not be easy

Even if all the participants who attend a group live under the same roof (for instance, in a residential hostel) or know each other from encounters in the locality, the fact that the joint group activity and the bond which takes time to establish is coming to an end will cause feelings associated with ending, similar to those of bereavement (see section 5.3). Depending on the clients' past experiences of separation, the feelings may include sadness, distress, anger or denial.

Prepare for the end

If you prepare your clients for the end, you will soften its impact. You can do this in various ways, depending on the kind of group you are running and on your clients. It is sensible to introduce the subject of the group's ending several sessions before the end, so that your clients are given time to come to terms with their feelings and to learn to accept that the group, like every encounter in life, has its end. Again, depending on the kind of group, you might wish to use the last session to help the clients express their feelings about the group experience. You can do this either in an informal discussion or by preparing a short questionnaire (which need not be signed so that the clients feel free to say whatever they wish). This will also give you valuable information about the way you ran the group, which you can then use for similar programmes in the future.

Encourage new relationships

Finally, encourage your clients to maintain friendships established during the group's meetings and outside it. One way of doing this is to encourage them to visit the drop-in centre (if there is one in your care setting or locality) where they can meet on neutral ground to deepen their friendship. You can also encourage them, if appropriate, to continue in private with the activity they learned in your group. For instance, a client might invite one or two others to his own home so that he can cook them a meal he learned during the cookery group. Remember, helping your clients to develop and maintain new relationships is a very important aspect of mental health care. Even when it ends, your group can provide a bridge from loneliness to finding new companions and new meaning to life.

Informal group activities

Although every group activity and every session has a planning and recruitment stage, and a beginning, middle and end, you are likely to be involved in less formal group work with clients as well.

ACTIVITY

1 Ask colleagues to help you make a chart listing informal group activities which took place in or outside your care setting during the past year. Leave space against each of these to list problems which occurred, if any. An extract from such a chart is given on the opposite page.

2 Drawing on your knowledge gained from this chapter, as well as suggestions from senior colleagues, list or discuss ways in which you could ensure that similar problems do not happen in the future.

Chart for group activities

March 1996 to March 1997		
Month and group activity	What happened	Future prevention
March: Local cinema (film)	S. (a client) over-reacted to an incident of rape in the film and caused a disturbance	Find out about the film and check the clients' personal histories (e.g. rape) in their case notes before the outing; inform the clients about the film's content
April: Party at the centre celebrating birthdays of four residents born this month	Someone brought a bottle of Scotch, and three clients were found drunk in the toilets	Clarify and establish boundaries regarding the agency's policy on drinking and make sure the clients know the consequences of breaking them; monitor parties more carefully, have more staff on duty
April: Quiz competition; general knowledge	All went well – our team won	

5 Supporting clients through personal difficulties

5.1 Supporting people in distress

All of us experience personal difficulties at some points in our lives. At such times we need understanding, acceptance and the support of those around us, whether it is emotional or practical. If we do not have the right kind of support when we need it, we might end up having mental health problems. This is because our psychological defence mechanism, which helps us to cope with stress, can be overloaded so that it breaks down. To stop this happening, you should give clients the right kind of support during personal difficulties.

Forms of distress

You will already be familiar with some forms of distress. It can be caused by:

- bereavement;
- personal trauma caused by a range of events such as divorce, infidelity of a partner or serious illness of a partner;
- terminal illness;
- worry about the future, one's job, health or children;
- shock at receiving bad news or shock due to an accident;
- a mental health condition, leading to psychological distress (including self-harm);
- frustration, leading to aggression and violence;
- sudden change of circumstances, such as unemployment;
- physical or emotional abuse;
- self-abuse, as in alcohol and drug abuse;
- problems in physical communication or other physical or sensory difficulties (for example, impaired hearing or vision).

ACTIVITY

1 What forms of distress do you think the clients in your care setting might be experiencing? Note down as many as you are aware of.

2 Now look into the case histories of two clients. Note down any events from their past which, in your opinion or the recorded opinion of other professionals, are likely to have caused prolonged stress or pain, or a feeling of failure or rejection.

ACTIVITY

Read the following two case studies, then answer the questions below.

Case study A

Mr Joseph Flint recently lost his business and became bankrupt. His sense of failure led to his hospitalisation, after which he was placed in your care setting. Recently he has heard from his daughter that his wife has been asking for a divorce so that she may remarry. Mr Flint feels extreme distress at having to lose his wife as well, not long after losing his business.

Case study B

Mrs Grace Walker lives alone in warden-staffed housing. On returning home one day, she unlocks her front door to get in when a man runs up behind her, pushes her inside and follows her in. She tries to scream, but he puts his hand over her mouth and proceeds to demand money and jewellery. He grabs her bag containing money and snatches her gold bracelet. Before leaving he attempts to rape her. The attempt fails as he hears a noise outside and escapes in a rush, leaving Mrs Walker in a state of shock.

1 You are a key worker for the clients in the above case studies. How would you go about helping each client with his or her distress?

2 Would you involve other people as well – professionals or the clients' relatives, for example? If yes, whom?

Ways of reducing distress

Mr Flint (Case study A) experienced distress when he lost his business and his wife, which brought him loss of income, social status and loss of companionship. All this will have a negative effect on his self-esteem. He could be helped by being counselled by a trained professional, but you can also provide direct support – refer to the previous parts of this book which dealt with self-esteem, communication, and listening and supporting skills (particularly sections 2.5 and 3.3).

Mrs Walker (Case study B) would benefit from your calm reassuring presence, especially because her home and privacy have been invaded and violated by an intruder. It might take some time for her to regain her lost feelings of personal safety, so the supportive worker must have patience. In cases of attack on a person, you will often have to involve people from outside your agency (see below).

Support from outside the agency

No matter how calm and sympathetic you are, just listening may not be sufficient. You should also act promptly. This may involve summoning help from outside your agency, such as:

- calling the client's doctor to examine for injuries or help the client deal with extreme distress;
- telephoning, writing or visiting anyone else whom the client wishes – her friend or a relative, for instance;
- contacting other agencies and organisations. In cases of distress caused by criminal action you should inform the police, but check this with the client and your supervisor first. You could also offer the client further befriending by contacting the local Victim Support agency.

ACTIVITY

1 Get in touch with your nearest Victim Support agency. Ask for information on the work they do.

2 Ask your supervisor if you could invite a speaker from Victim Support to talk to clients in your care setting about their work.

Practical or financial help

If, for example, the client has lost all her available cash, you should explore ways of helping her financially until her next payment arrives – perhaps by finding out about loans or using the amenity funds in your centre. Referring back to Case study B, Mrs Walker might feel intense fear at the thought of sleeping in the flat where the intrusion took place, so you might be asked to find temporary accommodation for her with relatives, friends, or in a hostel or bed and breakfast.

Distress within a care setting

A residential setting can be a stressful environment any time of day or night, whether you are a client or a worker. A day centre, too, can have its disturbances, as people get together to share their anxieties and worries. Sometimes over-reaction to everyday events occurs, because a client's coping mechanism is not as strong as that of an individual whose mental health is intact. The main task here would be to give a distressed person the opportunity to sit in a quiet and private place with a cup of tea and to speak to her in a calm and supportive manner.

Record keeping

Remember to make a written entry in the client's file for any incident which has caused significant distress to her. You might also want to inform colleagues at a staff meeting or sooner, so that they can act in a supporting role for the client when you are off duty.

Check your role

The ways in which incidents and crises are dealt with in a care setting, and by whom, depend on the nature of the agency. Check with your supervisor whenever you are not sure of your role.

Seek support for yourself

Your work requires you to act in a crisis with a cool and collected attitude. But you are not expected to be superhuman or to remain unaffected by such incidents. Once the worst is over and you are no longer expected to take the responsibility for your clients, you can be yourself again and try to relax. This means being aware of what you are experiencing in order to deal with the impact which the distressful incident might have had on you.

Burn-out

If you attempt to play down your own reactions to your clients' distress or to their destructive emotions and behaviour (see section 5.2), the stress will accumulate and manifest itself in various ways. You may find yourself gradually becoming fed up or depressed about your work; or perhaps cynical and less sensitive to your clients' needs. This is a natural defence, a psychological mechanism by which parts of our psyche guard against being hurt and affected by the difficulties, pains and misfortunes of others. The cumulative effect of stress and ignored negative emotions at work can result in a condition called burn-out, which is more common in the caring professions than is often recognised. Burn-out can also be shown by tiredness, sleeplessness, an increase of alcohol consumption, or a range of psychosomatic health problems in which your physical disorder is regarded as having a psychological basis.

Talk to someone

The symptoms of burn-out tend to develop in such a way that you yourself will usually be the last person to be aware of what is actually happening to you. That is why it is of absolute importance that you talk to someone as soon as possible after you have been through an emotionally demanding episode. Ask to see your supervisor or talk to a colleague.

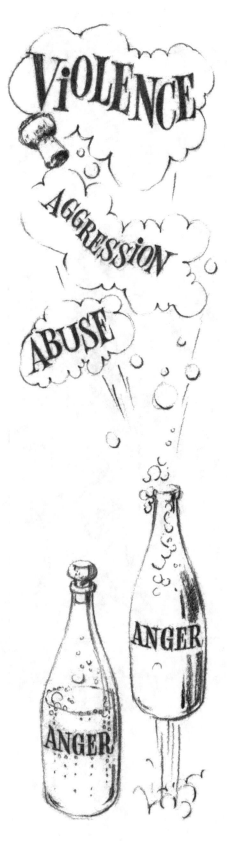

5.2 Dealing with distress resulting from aggression and violence

Distress as frustration and anger

Frustration and anger are valid and normal emotional reactions to have under certain conditions. But, as for other feelings, the longer anger is repressed, the more chance it has of erupting in unexpected situations and in less controllable ways.

When does anger become aggression?

This is sometimes a matter of individual or cultural interpretation. If you have spent all of your life in a social environment where there were no raised voices, you are more likely to experience a loud, angry encounter as distressing and aggressive. For another person it might be a normal part of everyday living.

   As a general guide, anger is an expression of feelings which does not have either a threat or abuse element. This does not mean that you do not feel a threat or apprehension caused by the angry person. But the point is that the person expressing anger does not make open threats, insult you, or physically harm you. When these things do happen, you are experiencing aggression.

ACTIVITY

1   Recall your most recent experience of seeing someone angry at work – a colleague or a client. Describe in short sentences or key phrases what actually happened.

2   Now do the same for the most recent incident of aggression or violence. If you have not witnessed one at work, ask a colleague to describe his or her impression of such an incident.

3   List the key differences. For example, observe the tone and volume of voice, language used, body movements and body language, and behaviour of the angry or aggressive person.

Aggression and violence

Some behaviours are so clear that most of us will react with fear and caution if we are near a person who expresses them. This could be when a person:

- hits an object such as a table with his fist or kicks a chair;
- shouts abuse or swears;
- expresses a verbal threat of violence;
- shows aggression towards the belongings of the individual he is angry with: for example, throws her handbag across the room;
- kicks, pushes or pulls at someone;
- employs various objects to hurt someone, such as a knife, gun or umbrella;
- uses provocation and menacing looks and gestures;
- employs racist or sexist language directed at his victim;
- is engaged in sexual aggression and violence, such as the use of unacceptable sexual language, touching, exposure, rape or its attempt.

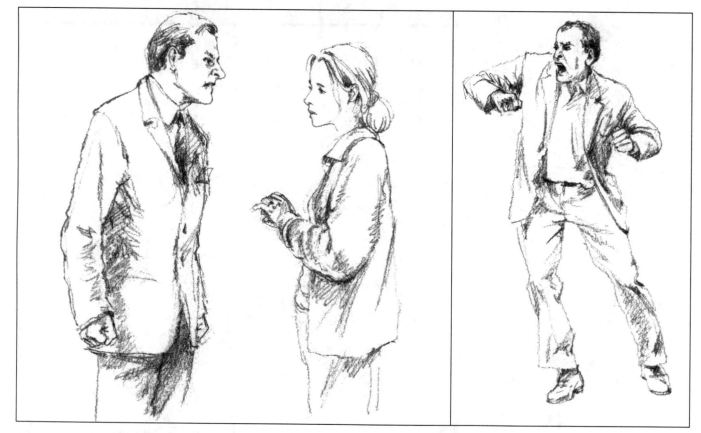

Aggression and violence take many different forms

What is achieved by aggression and violence?

People are aggressive and violent for different reasons; the main ones, though, are that such behaviour:

- gives a release to frustration;
- defends personal identity and self-worth: the victim is perceived by the aggressor as someone who represents danger to his self-esteem;
- defends and maintains external status, such as a macho image in front of others or the image of being a leader;

- brings about exploitation of others by using force and fear;
- satisfies a sadistic tendency, as in bullying and abuse;
- satisfies a need to control others and feel power over them; the basis for this need is personal insecurity.

Signs to watch out for

Non-verbal:

- clenched fists;
- restlessness, agitation;
- staring at a person, in eyeball-to-eyeball confrontation;
- provocative or threatening gestures;
- invasion of personal space;
- banging on an object, such as a wall or table.

Verbal:

- raised voice, higher pitch;
- very quiet, controlled threatening voice;
- language that is foul, racist or sexist;
- verbal threats;
- ritualistic repetition ('I have been here long enough and I want to be seen now, I want to be seen now, I told you I want to be seen now . . . I shan't tell you again, I want to be seen now');
- verbal address which is inappropriate – that is, not related to reality or showing psychological disturbance. For example, a client calls you by someone else's name and that person is his enemy, or says you are plotting against him with the FBI so he will get you.

Avoiding sticky situations

- Do not stand too close to someone who is agitated and showing signs of aggression.
- Do not stare at the angry person, but make intermittent eye-contact.
- Do not argue with an angry person as this will fuel the anger.
- A person who is about to lash out at someone can sometimes be distracted by, for example, an offer of a cup of tea.
- Do not think that you should be able to deal with a sticky situation on your own; calling a colleague to help does not suggest your failure but your common sense.
- Never reveal your home address to your clients.
- Learn how to restrain someone physically, if this is practised within your care setting. Learn your agency's policy on restraint. A course on basic self-defence skills will not be helpful unless you practise regularly, but it could increase your self-confidence which will help you remain calm and collected during those sticky moments.

Home visits to clients

Always tell colleagues or leave a message saying where you are going and what time you are expecting to be back. If visiting a client who is known to be potentially difficult, ask a colleague to accompany you.

How to handle aggression

When a client is known to you, it is easier to predict his or her behaviour. If, for instance, a client who frequently gets aggressive towards staff needs to be told some unpleasant news or needs to be confronted, you should ask these questions:

Who would be the best person to speak to the client?
It might be you if you have a good rapport with the client, or it might be a colleague. Or perhaps the client will respond better to a worker of the opposite gender.

Where?
If other clients are present, privacy seems a better option; but you should ensure that other workers are within close reach and that they are aware of what is going on. Always observe safety procedures; if you work with a client who is known to be violent, make sure you know where the emergency (panic) button is, and that you are sitting close to it and near the door. The environment should be clear of any objects which could be used as weapons or missiles.

When?
Timing is important. If you know that the client has had a frustrating day at the hospital, you might want to postpone the unpleasant 'chat' – provided, of course, that it isn't urgent.

ACTIVITY

1 Find out your care team's policy on dealing with clients who use abusive language such as swearing, racist or sexist comments.

2 Find out what sorts of things expressed by a client whose aggression is known to be due to her psychological condition are tolerated within your agency. What are its policy and guidelines to workers on unacceptable behaviour?

ACTIVITY

Ask several colleagues (preferably three) to join in this role play. Alternatively, this can be a group exercise in which most participants can observe.

Let one participant assume the role of a client who is abusive towards another client. You are the worker arriving on the scene, acting as you see fit. A senior colleague or supervisor should act as an observer.

After the role play, discuss:

- how you think you handled the situation;
- what you think, in retrospect, you could or should have done or said differently;

- what you think you need to learn (e.g. a particular aspect of the agency's policy) in order to feel more confident in the future.

Then ask the 'aggressor' what he or she thought of your action. Finally, the observer should give his comment.

By changing the roles and by enacting different incidents – some of which might include restraining clients, if this is practised in your care setting – this exercise can be used to provide training for the whole care team in how to deal with violence and aggression.

Psychological distress

Aggression and violence caused by mental health disturbance are far rarer than is popularly believed. However, they exist; clients who experience a relapse of their condition, especially the symptoms known as *paranoid schizophrenia*, can act violently. As the term 'paranoid' suggests, the client might experience an intense fear, usually about something which does not exist. When he attacks someone under such conditions, he believes he does this in self-defence or to fulfil his mission.

Signs

The main signs indicating a relapse are agitation and confused thinking with expression of violent intent, or reports of 'hearing voices' which the client might say are instructing her to act. These symptoms are easily controlled by medication, so acting promptly by calling a doctor is important.

Protect clients from aggression and violence

All care workers should be alert to any signs that suggest that clients are being exploited, victimised, bullied or sexually abused. Often the victim is afraid to report abuse for fear of being punished by the aggressor, or for fear of losing his 'only friend', which the aggressor might seem to be. Talking to such clients confidentially and educating them on what is appropriate behaviour and what is not can help. Teaching them to be assertive and express their wishes clearly and confidently might take time, but it is effort well spent.

Report the aggressor's behaviour

Report any incident of abuse of a client by another client to your supervisor and senior colleagues. Record the incident, following your agency's procedure, as soon as you can. Also report and try to collect evidence if you suspect that the aggressor might be someone other than client, perhaps the client's friend, a family member, or a member of staff.

Aggressors and abusers need support too

When you really know all about someone, their childhood, their fears and concerns, you can usually understand why the person is acting in a particular manner. Your desire to understand the behaviour of an aggressor does not mean that you condone the behaviour. If you look at the behaviour and the person as separate things, you will be able to give support to a client who has been abusing others or committing acts of violence. When such clients are willing to change, they could be offered professional counselling.

Self-abuse by alcohol or drugs

Alcohol and drug abuse should be dealt with promptly, and every agency should have a clear policy on this. Clients who have become dependent on these substances need specialised professional help. You can help by talking to them about their options, and supporting them when they accept such help.

Aggression from colleagues

In a survey reported in *Community Care*, April 1995, social workers said that they experienced far more stress at work from their colleagues than from clients. Perhaps because workers are expected to be caring towards clients all the time, they need to compensate by being the opposite to each other!

Although workers aim to be caring and fair in all their dealings, social care can be dominated by the desire for power. We live in a highly competitive society, so do not get disillusioned at the first experience of bullying or being criticised. But do not submit to it either if you are sure that the criticism is not valid.

Be firm

If you are experiencing bullying or other forms of aggression or assault from a colleague, be firm in telling the person that you will not tolerate such behaviour. If the aggression persists, one way of dealing with the problem is to ask another colleague to act as an observer. When you have some concrete evidence and someone to support you, you will be able to proceed with reporting the aggressor to a higher authority.

Of course, you could, and whenever possible should, go to your supervisor right away and complain, but this will only help if you have a very good rapport with her – that is, if she values you at least as much as the aggressor. Otherwise it is your word against the bully's, who may be someone of a higher professional status than you.

Sometimes care team managers fail to recognise problems among staff; perhaps because they are overworked or because they are unable to deal with problems of staff relationships and group dynamics (see section 4.5). In such cases, be prepared to collect evidence so that you can go to a higher authority.

> **ACTIVITY**
>
> **1** Speak to *approved social workers* (see section 1.5) about their dealings with clients who are aggressive or violent because of distress caused by their mental health. What do they advise you should do if you find yourself alone with such clients?
>
> **2** Find out whom, if anyone, you could talk to at work if you felt exposed to aggression and abuse by a client. Can you talk to someone if the aggressor is a member of staff?

Caring does not mean tolerating abuse

Some workers believe that being tolerant of verbal aggression and abuse by clients is part of being caring. Some clients use their mental health status in a manipulative way; they abuse others and then excuse themselves by saying their behaviour was a symptom of their mental health. Racist and sexist behaviours are often excused in this way. Sometimes staff accept this because they are afraid of causing more distress to the aggressor by confronting the behaviour. The result is a repetition of the unacceptable behaviour, harmful to both clients and workers.

This should not be so. You and your colleagues deserve respect and the freedom to work without fearing aggressive clients or colleagues, or hearing their insults. Get help if you are experiencing abuse. If you cannot get help from your colleagues, which should always be your first option, look for support outside.

For your information

★ If you are experiencing bullying or other forms of abuse at work (e.g. racial or sexual harassment) and you fear the possible consequences, such as loss of your job, of revealing it to your employer, you can ask for confidential legal advice from the following organisation: Public Concern at Work, Lincoln's Inn House, 42 Kingsway, London WC2B 6EN.

Further reading

★ *The ABC of Handling Aggression* by Willie More, published by Pepar Publications in 1993 (third edition), is a readable book written for social care workers.

5.3 Supporting clients at times of loss

In Chapter 1 (section 1.2) references were made to events which most people find stressful. There is evidence to suggest that most people who have mental health problems have experienced a higher number of these events than other people. Most, though not all, of these events involve some kind of loss: the loss of someone (e.g. a partner or child, for instance) or of something (e.g. job, health, home, privacy or money).

Loss of someone – bereavement

Bereavement follows every significant loss, whether through separation, divorce or death. Those left behind need time to mourn the loss and readjust to life without the person who has gone or died. Clients need to be supported during this period with all the available skills and resources, because successful grieving can prevent further mental health difficulties.

Support during bereavement

Do

- Give clients your time, but also be sensitive when they want privacy.
- Allow each individual to express grief in her or his own way.
- Encourage sharing thoughts and reminiscing.
- Show that you can imagine and feel some of their pain – show empathy. For example, you could say 'You really hurt, don't you?' or 'It must be very painful to lose someone you felt so close to.'

Expressing feelings about the loss
Encourage clients to express different emotions concerning the loss. These could be sadness and grief, loneliness, confusion or helplessness. Be aware that they may be trying to hide their true feelings because of the fear of being judged. These could be anger, perhaps because of the feeling of being deserted, or relief if the client had to endure a long and difficult time while caring for the deceased. Guilt is a common reaction, while ambivalent relationships could leave resentment, or perhaps even joy if the client felt trapped in a relationship in which she was abused. Asking the client 'What will you miss about him least?' or 'What won't you miss?' is a gentle way to encourage the voicing of these feelings.

Helping to consolidate the reality of the loss
If the client deliberately avoids the subject of the loss, which is a sign of denial, gently introduce the subject. You can help him to accept reality by asking questions about the circumstances of the loss and about the funeral.

Encouraging – giving realistic hope
Give encouragement when the client despairs. Reassure him that he will feel better in time, but that the memories of the loved one will always live on. Be careful not to do this right at the beginning, however; you should help the client to acknowledge the loss first and allow him to express feelings about it.

ACTIVITY

If you have had the misfortune of losing someone close to you, you can do this activity using your personal experience; otherwise imagine that someone very close to you has died.

1 Write down the kinds of comments, conversations or behaviour of others you did or would find helpful.

2 What was or would be unhelpful?

Don't

- Do not avoid the client or the topic of her loss. If you find that you are avoiding such conversations, ask yourself why. If the client's loss has triggered memories and distress of your own past losses, speak to your supervisor about it, and perhaps a counsellor as well.
- Never talk about your own or other people's losses to the client. She is the one who needs support from you, not vice versa.
- Do not minimise the client's loss by saying, for example, 'Everybody loses their parents, it's normal.' Although true in general, this does not lessen the significance of each individual's loss.

It was only a dog – why not get another?

Do not underestimate the effect which a loss of a pet can have on some individuals. For someone living alone, such a loss can be as significant as the loss of a human counterpart. Time for grieving is needed here, too. Although you can never replace a lost friend or partner, you can have someone new later, once you have grieved and become ready to reinvest your feelings and energy; the same goes for losing a pet.

Let's cheer you up...

Do not try to cheer up the client by making jokes or arranging other entertainment for her when she is clearly not ready to participate.

You're so morbid...

Never say that talking about the circumstances of the death is 'morbid'. Sometimes people need to recall these over and over again. This will help the reality of the loss to sink in, especially when the initial response might have been disbelief, shock or numbness.

Religion can help you...

Do not try to comfort clients with your own religious beliefs – 'She must be in heaven now', for instance – but respect their religious faith or lack of it.

You should be over her by now...

Never tell a client that he has grieved long enough. There is no prescribed time for the grieving process.

Cultural aspects of bereavement

Every culture has its own customs in respect to death and mourning. It is important, therefore, that you respect the client's choice regarding the rituals of burial and mourning. The same applies for the anniversaries. If your agency is responsible for the practical arrangements of the funeral, the cultural and religious aspects should be honoured as much as possible.

Other kinds of loss

Similar feelings can be experienced by other kinds of loss, such as the loss of a job through redundancy or retirement, the loss of a child by means other than death, as for example by adoption, or the loss of a partner through separation or divorce. Self-esteem suffers greatly in these sorts of loss. The

---

ACTIVITY

If you work in a multicultural care setting, ask colleagues or clients from different cultures to describe to you the customs of burial and the social and religious aspects of mourning. Do this for up to three cultures.

If you work in a monocultural setting, you may have friends from different cultures who could supply such information. If not, find the relevant information in your local library.

sense of failure and guilt can be so intense that the person might even contemplate taking his or her own life. Be sensitive to what the loss means to each client: never make assumptions about it.

Suicide

Death by suicide is a very difficult form of loss for people to come to terms with. The feelings of guilt and failure are immense, so the bereaved will need a lot of support.

Prevention

It is easy for clients to accumulate medication, by not taking tablets regularly or telling their doctor they have accidentally lost their pills and so getting more. A residential setting is easier to check for the accumulation of pills, but even here it is not possible to keep track of all objects and substances which a client could use for self-harm. The best prevention is the emotional and social support given to clients who are depressed, offering them hope that life will get better.

Your client has taken his own life

If the client for whom you have been a key worker has taken his own life, you should talk about your feelings to your supervisor or a colleague. Care workers often blame themselves and feel they should have seen it coming, visited the client earlier, alerted the client's doctor, or searched his room for signs of accumulation of tablets. But remember, no one can be responsible for someone 24 hours a day, no matter how caring he or she is.

Forgive yourself for being human

You always care as well as you can at any given time; judging yourself with hindsight is pointless. It is like saying that you do not permit yourself to be human, have limitations or make mistakes.

Whatever you do, do not bottle up your feelings (see section 5.1). Find out what resources your care setting has to help their workers with stresses brought about at work, so that you know what to do when you need help.

ACTIVITY

1   Find out details of your local branch of CRUSE (a voluntary organisation which provides bereavement counselling – see Appendix 2) and make enquiries so that you know how you can refer a client for counselling, how long the waiting list is, and other key details.

2   Find out about agencies offering bereavement counselling for people who have a terminal illness.

3   Try to trace a self-help group for relatives and friends of suicide victims. Can any of your clients benefit from attending it?

For your information

★   The Samaritans have made a video, *Always There*, which addresses the problem of suicide among young people. Look in your local telephone directory for the local branch of The Samaritans.

5.4 Helping people towards independent living

Clients' dependency on your care setting should never be viewed as indefinite. Although you must accept that some individuals will always need help, even they can reduce their level of dependency.

Independence in a residential setting

When clients no longer need the high levels of support that are typically provided in a mental health residential setting – often around the clock, when staff have sleep-in duties or stay on duty till bedtime – it is time for them to move on. It makes sense to make the move gradual, so many agencies arrange for these clients to have homes, whether individual flats or sharing with others, close to the residential setting. This is beneficial for two reasons. First, the same staff can give clients support during the early days of independent living; second, clients can continue to visit their former home and keep in touch with friends and other residents.

There may be other routes to independence. For example, a client may go to live with her family or move to another area closer to it, or she may marry someone or live with a partner who becomes the carer as well.

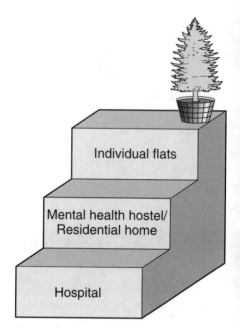

Stairs of independence

ACTIVITY

1 What is the longest period that a client has been receiving help from your agency? What has kept the client dependent for so long?

2 Find out from colleagues about clients who no longer come for support to your care setting. What has happened to them? Where are they living? What are they doing?

3 Think of clients who have recently become more independent; perhaps they moved into their own flat, got a job, or went on to do training. For each of them, list things which, in your opinion, helped them to arrive where they are now.

Independence begins in your care setting

You cannot expect clients who have not acted independently – cooked for themselves, done the shopping or made decisions – for a long time to suddenly be able to do these things when they are left on their own. This is why independence should start in a care setting, where it is sometimes related to client empowerment – workers enabling and allowing clients to take over aspects of care which they are capable of.

What can clients do?

Generally this will depend mainly on what services and activities are provided by your agency and for what kind of clients – that is, according to the state of their mental health as well as physical abilities.

ACTIVITY

1 List the ways in which clients in your agency participate in activities and decision making associated with their care.

2 Discuss with your colleagues and supervisor your ideas on how the level of clients' participation can be improved.

3 Why do you think that clients should participate in their own care?

Decision making on some level should be the most important part of preparing clients for independent living. For example, clients can decide:

- where the centre's annual holiday should take place (taking account of available funds);
- how to make fair and democratic decisions about who will go on a subsidised holiday when there is a limited number of places;
- where to go for day trips and how (mode of transport);
- which newspapers should be bought for clients to read at the centre, or which books;
- how to spend funds given for improvement of their residential home;
- whether to participate in activities in the local community such as annual fairs;
- how to raise money;
- about the menu for their meals or snacks.

They are likely to need some help from care workers in making decisions; the level of help will depend on the clients' ability to decide or do things on their own. They will, however, often need information and co-operation from carers: for example, how much money the centre has available for outings.

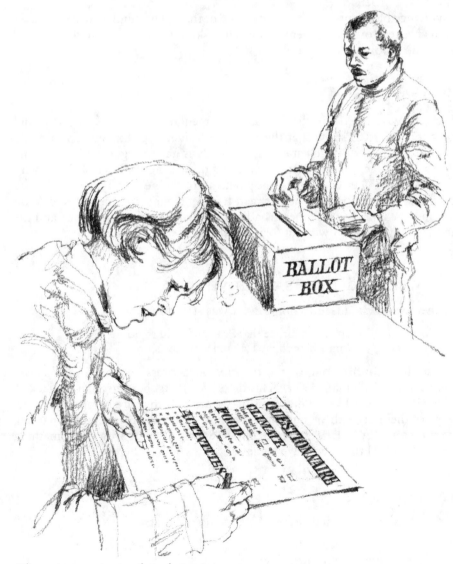

Clients communicating their choices

Practical tasks

Clients can be involved in doing a variety of practical tasks such as:

- helping make the care environment a pleasant place to be in, for example by keeping it tidy and clean, caring for the pot plants and gardening;
- welcoming newcomers and showing them around;
- providing assistance to staff during special occasions, such as food preparation for Christmas dinner or ethnic festivals, or shopping for goods for the centre;
- making enquiries about outings, booking tickets for the cinema, or arranging transport for a day trip;
- helping in creative activities such as preparation of the agency's newsletter or creating posters and information sheets for various events organised by the centre.

A more independent client can act as a befriender to a vulnerable client during hospital visits or shopping trips.

Opportunity to work – not servitude

Involving able clients in light work should be therapeutic and help them master skills needed for independent living. They should never be treated as unpaid or cheap labour.

Work schemes

If clients wish to do a particular task on a regular basis, some reward would be appropriate to show that their work is valued. For example, you could create a clients' work scheme for tasks such as gardening, cleaning, making and selling snacks in the drop-in, mending or making clothes or helping with a jumble sale. They could get some payment for their effort, but you will need to check with the benefits department for clients who are unemployed or on sickness benefit, because there is a limit to the hours they can work and the money they can earn without losing their usual state payments.

Why should clients do anything?

In the poem *Listen* (see section 3.3), it was stated that:

> When you do something for me that I can and need to do
> for myself, you contribute to my fear and weakness.

These lines confirm one of the theories on depression known as *learned helplessness* (Seligman, 1975). This theory suggests that, through the lack of control over their lives, individuals may learn that they are helpless, and this view of themselves then contributes to their feeling depressed and remaining so as long as they feel they have no control. So when clients are given something to do, they feel that they have some control, which is therapeutic.

Other reasons

Other reasons for giving clients things to do are that:

- it makes them feel useful, which is good for their self-esteem;
- it gives structure to their day;

ACTIVITY

1 If you know clients in your care setting who are presently helping to do tasks either in or outside your agency, list what, in your opinion, they are gaining by it?

2 Why do you think clients who are able should do practical tasks?

- it recreates a sense of responsibility which has been damaged because of mental health difficulties and, often, institutionalisation;
- it can lead to new social relationships;
- it can help them feel they are active members of a care unit and not mere recipients of care.

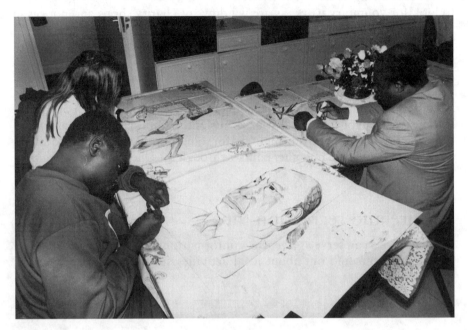

An art group

What clients need for independent living

Once you are sure that clients have the skills necessary to move on, you need to check the following aspects of their new lives:

- *accommodation*: this must be arranged *before* the client leaves the care setting to prevent homelessness;
- *finance* for food, shelter, bills, clothes and leisure (see section 3.5);
- *continuing mental health care*: check-ups with the doctor, depot clinic attendance or attendance of psychotherapy groups;
- *physical health*: for example, support to clients pending an operation;
- *liaison with other workers* to ensure that the client does not lose contact with care professionals such as OTs (occupational therapists), CPNs (community psychiatric nurses), GPs, and social workers;
- *family contact*: ensuring that the client's family is involved whenever possible, recognising that for some clients this might be counterproductive;
- *daytime occupation*: ensuring that the client is not left with nothing to do by exploring employment (voluntary or paid), training and educational opportunities, or attendance at activities in day centres in the locality;
- *social network*: clients should move to an area where it is easy for them to keep in touch with friends or meet new friends.

Employment

Support clients in their first attempt to return to work after a period of unemployment; they will need a confidence boost. Also help them to achieve self-discipline in getting up in the morning to arrive at work on time.

Voluntary work

This could provide a good way to gain skills and experience before seeking paid employment. Alternatively, if the work is enjoyed for its own sake, it can give fulfilment, while many kinds of volunteer jobs provide an opportunity for socialising as well. The notice board in a local library is a good place to look for voluntary work, as are windows of charity shops and notices in local papers. Most agencies pay expenses.

Training schemes

From time to time, voluntary organisations and charities run training schemes for different groups of people, including those with mental health problems. If these exist in your area, tell your clients and encourage them to attend.

Clients who have been unemployed for some months may qualify to attend a range of NVQ/SVQ and other courses through the Unemployment Training Office.

Leisure and recreation time

Local libraries can serve as a centre of information on training, studying and leisure. You can find out about local activities such as dramatic societies,

ACTIVITY

1 Get in touch with your local employment office and find out about the current training opportunities for unemployed clients. Display such information in your care setting.

2 Talk to clients who are showing signs of higher levels of independence about their aspirations, hopes and plans for future work, training or studying. Help them to find out more about their chosen field.

You do not have to leave your room to keep fit

poetry or creative writing groups, music groups (playing, singing or listening) and sports clubs. People with low incomes do not need to join expensive clubs for the sake of exercise or leisure; strolling along country lanes, jogging, cycling, or a brisk walk through a park in a city can be equally beneficial.

Look out for small changes

You might sometimes feel discouraged, especially when you work with clients who do not seem to make much progress or even become more dependent on carers. Do not view this as a measure of your efforts and contribution to their care. Even clients with a long-term and severe mental distress go through periods of hope and self-determination when they enjoy their lives. Look out for such moments closely, otherwise you may be left with a false impression that mental health care means gloom for most of the time.

Have fun

Some carers forget that clients, too, have a sense of humour – that they like to laugh, sing or dance. Encourage this whenever possible. For example, a group activity can include a regular outing to a dance or an informal singing session at the centre, especially if a client or a member of staff can play a musical instrument. And don't be afraid to laugh with clients or to try to make them laugh, when appropriate, because laughter is therapeutic: it is uplifting.

How to value your work

There will be times when you question the value of what you are trying to do. This is natural, especially when you see those you care for have a relapse over and over again, or when someone takes his own life, commits self-harm or harms someone else. Often carers' pain and feelings of failure are enhanced a hundredfold by media reports and accusations.

Such moments of doubts will come, and you must learn to accept them as part of your work. You must also learn to let go of them in order to channel all your energies into what you do.

To help you through these trying times, remember that you have chosen one of the most challenging fields of care. That choice in itself shows that you have the strength – though at times it may be hidden even from yourself – to carry on and learn from such situations.

Remember, too, that mental health care is made up of many small steps, and that many professionals will be involved in making the clients' journey to independence as comfortable as possible. As you learn to empathise with your clients, you will begin to value what you do through their eyes, rather than by having your own high (perhaps unrealistic) expectations for them. Share in their excitement and joy at the centre's outing, for example – remember, life is made up of such moments lived to the full.

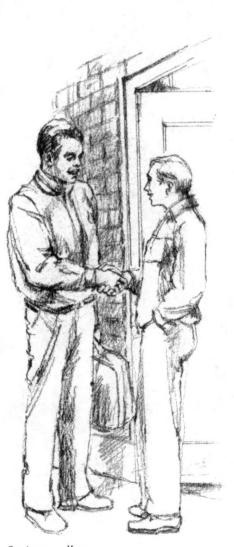

Saying goodbye

5.5 Evaluation: looking back and forwards

The aim of this final section is to enable you to test yourself on the knowledge and skills described in this workbook. It will also help you to become aware of any gaps in your knowledge, information and skills which are relevant to the requirements of the particular client group you are working for.

Answer the questions below. If you cannot think of the answers, go back to the section of the workbook indicated in order to revise your knowledge. Many questions here demand specific answers, but some do not. These are designed to help you pursue further knowledge, skill or creative ideas which will be of special value for your care setting.

Check with your supervisor or senior colleagues if you are not sure about your answers – but only after you have revised each section of the workbook.

Revision

Chapter 1

1 How can you and your colleagues help to change the public image of people with mental health problems? Give three suggestions. (Refer to section 1.1.)

2 Give six significant symptoms of depression. (Refer to section 1.2.)

3 Which of the following can be a side effect of taking an antidepressant? (Refer to section 1.2.)

   (a) sweating   (d) singing   (g) cardiac problems
   (b) limping   (e) drowsiness   (h) blurred vision
   (c) nausea   (f) rheumatism   (i) muscle twitching

4 Which of the following describes supervision registers? (Refer to section 1.4.)
   (a) Methods for managing and supervising staff in a care agency.
   (b) Registers used by professionals so that they can keep an eye on clients who live in the community.
   (c) Registers kept by supervisors for recording their observations of the work and professional development of staff whom they supervise.

5 Describe the meaning of the following terms. (Refer to section 1.4.)
   (a) provider of care
   (b) purchaser of care
   (c) care plan
   (d) case (care) manager

6 Which of the following can be achieved by application of the Mental Health Act 1983? (Refer to section 1.5.)
   (a) A client can sue her psychiatrist for administering medication against her will.
   (b) A carer can speed up the process of getting the local authorities to house her client.
   (c) A relative can make an application for a client to be taken into hospital by force.
   (d) A police constable can take a person who appears to be experiencing mental distress to the police station.
   (e) Mental health professionals can apply to the Minister of Health for a rise in their salaries.

Chapter 2

1 Name at least four kinds of settings where mental health care takes place, preferably in your locality. (Refer to section 2.1.)

2 Give a description of the key roles of each of the following care professionals. (Refer to section 2.1.)
   (a) community psychiatric nurse (CPN)
   (b) approved social worker
   (c) psychologist
   (d) psychiatrist

3 List at least three suitable ways of preparing for a meeting in your care setting, stating which meeting you have in mind. (Refer to section 2.2.)

4 What are the five stages which represent the process of caring for clients? (Refer to section 2.3.)

5 Draw a rough assessment interview guide which could be used as an aid to help you ask the right kind of questions during an assessment interview. (Refer to section 2.3.)

6 What assessment skills should a care worker possess? List as many as you can think of. (Refer to section 2.3.)

7 What kinds of information used in your care setting should be kept secure? (Refer to section 2.4.)

8 What non-verbal aspects of your behaviour can improve your communication with clients? How? (Refer to section 2.5.)

9 What aspects of cultural differences do you think you should know in order to offer better care to clients from other cultures in your locality? (Refer to section 2.6.)

10 Identify problems, if any, which you have (or might have) when caring for a person who has a different sexual orientation than your own. (Refer to section 2.7.)

11 State ways in which you could help others or yourself to overcome such problems. (Refer to section 2.7.)

12 What legislation exists to guard against discrimination made on racial, sexual, disability, age, health or other grounds? (Refer to section 2.8.)

Chapter 3

1 List eight duties of a key worker, ticking those which apply to your care setting. (Refer to section 3.1.)

2 How should you behave towards your clients in order to develop a good professional relationship with them? (Refer to section 3.2.)

3 What kinds of responses and behaviour should you avoid to show that you are an empathic listener? (Refer to section 3.3.)

4 Give two examples each of 'open' and 'closed' questions, indicating situations when you might use them. (Refer to section 3.4.)

5 Make a list of local services which can be of use to clients in your care setting. (Refer to section 3.5.)

6 Which living skills would clients in your care setting need to master before they could live more independent lives? (Refer to section 3.6.)

7 List precautions which you, your clients and your colleagues should take to ensure protection against the spread of viral infections. (Refer to section 3.7.)

8 Think of situations in which clients in mental health care might wish to have an advocate. (Refer to section 3.8.)

9 Give examples of questions which you might wish to ask the client during the process of reviewing your individual work with him or her. (Refer to section 3.9.)

Chapter 4

1 Name the most important benefits for clients when they participate in group activities provided by mental health carers. (Refer to section 4.1.)

2 What are some of the things you should consider and research when planning to set up a formal group activity? (Refer to section 4.2.)

3 List some of the objectives you should have when planning a group for clients in your care. (Refer to section 4.3.)

4 What questions should you ask yourself when planning a group? (Refer to section 4.4.)

5 Which tasks might fall within a group leader's role? (Refer to section 4.4.)

6 How would you go about helping a client who stands out from others during the group activity? Give suggestions for each of the following. (Refer to section 4.5.)
   (a) a client who has a different ethnic origin
   (b) a client who has a different sexual orientation
   (c) a client who has a physical disability (state which)

Chapter 5

1 What action might a carer take to help her client deal with distress caused by the following? (Refer to section 5.1.)
   (a) physical illness
   (b) loss of finance
   (c) verbal abuse by another client
   (d) physical abuse

2 Which non-verbal and which verbal signs should you watch out for when someone might become aggressive or violent? (Refer to section 5.2.)

3 List some things you should say or do to help a bereaved client mourn his or her loss. (Refer to section 5.3.)

4 What are the things you should not do? (Refer to section 5.3.)

5 Write a checklist which shows what skills a client with mental health difficulties might need for life in the community. You could use this list to help you prepare your clients for a greater level of independence. (Refer to section 5.4.)

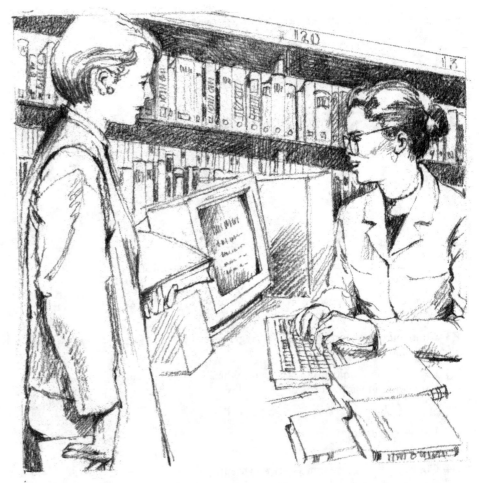

The library is a good source of information

Beyond the *Mental Health Care* workbook

Make a list of topics and skills which you need to learn and which were not covered in this workbook – perhaps because of the more specialised nature of your work or your course. Ask your supervisor, colleagues or a librarian whom you should contact (which organisations) and where you should look (which literature) to find out information that is not covered here.

Appendix 1:
Links to NVQs/ SVQs

Level 3 core units	Sections of this book
O Promote equality for all individuals	2.6, 2.7, 2.8
Z1 Contribute to the protection of individuals from abuse	2.5, 3.8, 5.2
Z3 Contribute to the management of aggressive and abusive behaviour	2.5, 5.2
Z4 Promote communication with clients when there are communication difficulties	2.6, 2.7, 3.3, 3.4, 4.5
Z8 Support clients when they are distressed	3.3, 3.7, 5.1, 5.2, 5.3
Y2 Enable clients to make use of available services and information	2.3, 2.4, 3.5, 3.8, 5.4
U4 Contribute to the health, safety and security of individuals and their environment	1.4, 2.5, 3.1, 3.3, 3.6, 3.7, 5.2
U5 Obtain, transmit and store information relating to the delivery of a care service	2.3, 2.4, 3.9, 4.5

Mental health care endorsement	Sections of this book
Z2 Contribute to the provision of advocacy for clients	3.8
X2 Prepare and provide agreed individual development activities for clients	2.3, 3.1, 3.6, 5.4
X16 Prepare and implement agreed therapeutic group activities	4.1, 4.2, 4.3, 4.4, 4.5
W1 Support clients in developing their identity and personal relationships	1.2, 2.6, 2.7, 2.8, 3.2, 3.3, 4.5
W5 Support clients with difficult or potentially difficult relationships	2.5, 2.6, 2.7, 3.3, 3.8, 5.2
W8 Enable clients to maintain contacts in potentially isolating situations	4.1, 4.5, 5.4

Other level 3 units	Sections of this book
Z14 Support clients and others at times of loss	5.3
Z18 Support individuals where abuse has been disclosed	5.1, 5.2
Y3 Enable clients to administer their financial affairs	3.5, 3.6
Y5 Assist clients to move from a supportive to an independent living environment	3.5, 3.6, 5.4

Level 2 and 3 unit	Sections of this book
V1 Contribute to the planning and monitoring of service delivery	1.4, 2.2, 2.3, 2.4, 3.1, 3.9, 4.4, 4.5

Level 2 unit	Sections of this book
Z13 Enable clients to participate in recreation and leisure activities	4.3, 5.4

Appendix 2: Useful contacts

There is not enough space here to list all the many organisations which exist within mental health fields; you will find details of some at the end of sections within the book which deal with specific concerns. Some organisations, especially those offering self-help, move premises fairly frequently as they have no permanent premises. Please check their details before you give them to your clients or their relatives.

Mental health organisations and societies

Many of the organisations listed here offer information, including free leaflets on various issues concerning mental health, while some offer training to workers as well as counselling, support and other help to the clients. They can also supply details of useful similar organisations in your locality.

Ex-services Mental Welfare Society, Broadway House, The Broadway, London SW19 1RL. Tel. 0181 543 6333. For Scotland, Ireland, Isle of Man and Northern England: Hollybush House, Hollybush By Ayr KA60 7EA. Tel. 01292 560 214.

Glasgow Association for Mental Health (GAMH), 1st Floor, Melrose House, 15/23 Cadogen Street, Glasgow G2 6QQ. Tel. 0141 204 2270.

Mental Health Task Force, Department of Health, Richmond House, London SW1A 2NS. Tel. 0171 210 4850.

MIND, 15–19 Broadway, London E15 4BQ. Tel. 0181 519 2122.

Richmond Fellowship Scotland, 9 Sandyford Place, Glasgow G3 7NB. Tel. 0141 248 4818.

Scottish Association for Mental Health (SAMH), Atlantic House, 38 Gardner's Crescent, Edinburgh EH3 8DQ. Tel. 0131 229 9687/228 5185.

Counselling – psychotherapy

Most agencies listed below offer a free counselling service, although some (e.g. BAC) may ask for a small contribution, often depending on your income.

British Association for Counselling (BAC), 1 Regent Place, Rugby, Warwickshire CV21 2PJ. Tel. 01788 578328.

Counsel and Care, Twyman House, 16 Bonny Street, London NW1 9PG. Tel. 0171 485 1550.

CRUSE (Bereavement Care), 126 Sheen Street, Richmond, Surrey TW9 1UR. Tel. 0181 940 4818.

Gay and Lesbian Switchboard (Central Office, ask for local groups), Tel. 0171 837 7324.

National Aids Helpline, PO Box 5000, Glasgow G12 9JQ. Tel. 0800 567123.

No. 21 Counselling Service, 21 Rutland Square, Edinburgh EH1 2BB. Tel. 0131 221 9377.

RELATE (Relationship Counselling), Herbert Grey College, Little Church Street, Rugby, Warwickshire SV21 3AP. Tel. 01788 573241.

The Samaritans (Head Office in Slough), Tel. 01753 532713.

Women's Therapy Centre, 6 Manor Gardens, London N7 6LA. Tel. 0171 263 6200.

Multiracial counselling and information

Asian Family Counselling Service (Head Office), 2nd Floor, 40 Equity Chambers, Piccadilly, Bradford, West Yorkshire BD1 3NN. Tel. 01274 720486. Also 72 The Avenue, London W13 8LB. Tel. 0181 997 5749.

Chinese Information and Advice Centre, 68 Shaftesbury Avenue, London W1V 7DF. Tel. 0171 836 8291,

Unity Helpline (Multiracial counselling and information telephone service, and local referrals), 2–4 Ravenstone Street, Balham, London SW12 9SS. Tel. 0181 673 0793.

Self-help groups

There are groups for various forms of mental health problems which can be of help to clients, their relatives and friends. Mental health organisations (e.g. MIND) can supply other contacts.

Depressives Anonymous, 36 Chestnut Avenue, Beverley, North Humberside HU17 9QU. Tel. 01482 860619. Also 57 Moira Court, Trinity Crescent, London SW17 7AQ. Tel. 0181 767 1920.

ECT Anonymous, 14 Western Avenue, Riddlesden, Keighley, West Yorkshire BD20 5DJ. Tel. 01535 661493.

Gwynedd Users Forum, c/o MIND, 42 Glanrafon, Bangor, Gwynedd, North Wales. Tel. 01248 353777.

The Manic Depression Fellowship, 8–10 High Street, Kingston-upon-Thames, Surrey KT1 1EY. Tel. 0181 974 6550.

Narcotics Anonymous, PO Box 704, London SW10 0RN. Tel. 0171 730 0009.

National Hearing Voices Network, c/o Creative Support, Fourways House, Tariff Street, Manchester M1 2EP. Tel. 0161 288 3896.

Stresswatch, The Barn, 42 Barnweil Road, Riccarton, Kilnarnock KAI 4JF. Tel. 01563 574144.

Holistic healing

British Acupuncture Association, 34 Alderney Street, London SW1V 4EU. Tel. 0171 834 1012.

British Homoeopathic Association, 27a Devonshire Street, London W1N 1RJ. Tel. 0171 935 2163.

Education and training

Central Council for Education and Training in Social Work Information Service, Derbyshire House, St Chad's Street, London WC1 8AD. Tel. 0171 278 2455.

Community Care Group, King's Fund, 11–13 Cavendish Square, London W1M 0AN. Tel. 0171 307 2400.

HMSO Publications Centre (Mail and telephone orders), PO Box 276, London SW8 5DT. Tel. 0171 873 9090.

Open College, Freepost, PO Box 35, Abingdon, OX14 3BR.

Miscellaneous

Age Concern England, Astral House, 1268 London Road, London SW16 4EG. Tel. 0181 679 8000.

Alcohol Concern, Waterbridge House, 32–36 Loman Street, London SE1 0EE. Tel. 0171 928 7377.

British Medical Association, BMA House, Tavistock Square, London WC1H 9JP. Tel. 0171 387 4499.

Commission for Racial Equality (CRE), Elliott House, 10–12 Allington Street, London SW1E 5EH. Tel. 0171 828 7022.

Disabled Living Foundation, 380–384 Harrow Road, London W9 2HU. Tel. 0171 289 6111.

DSS Information Division (Leaflets Unit), Block 4, Government Buildings, Honeypot Lane, Stanmore, Middlesex HA7 1AY.

Health and Safety Executive, Rose Court, 2 Southwark Bridge, London SE1 9HS. Tel. 0171 717 6000.

Standing Conference on Drug Abuse (SCODA), Waterbridge House, 32–36 Loman Street, London SE1 0EE. Tel. 0171 928 9500.

Appendix 3: Bibliography

Beech, D. 1991. *Social Work and Mental Disorder*. Birmingham: PEPAR Publications.

BMA and RPSGB 1992. *British National Formulary*. London: British Medical Association and Pharmaceutical Press.

Burke, A. 1986. 'Racism, Prejudice and Mental Illness' in J. Cox (ed.) *Transcultural Psychiatry*. London: Croom Helm.

George, M. 1995. 'Study Reveals High Levels of Stress and Racism' in *Community Care*, 20–26 April 1995.

HMSO 1989. *Caring for People: Community Care in the Next Decade and Beyond*. London: Her Majesty's Stationery Office.

HMSO 1993. *Code of Practice, Mental Health Act 1983*. London: Her Majesty's Stationery Office.

HMSO 1994. *Mental Health Act 1983*. London: Her Majesty's Stationery Office.

Kitzinger, C. and Coyle, A. 1995. 'Lesbian and Gay Couples: Speaking of Differences' in *The Psychologist* 8, 64–9. Leicester: The British Psychological Society.

More, W. 1993. *The ABC of Handling Aggression* (third edition). Birmingham: PEPAR Publications.

Parry *et al.* 1981. 'Reliability of Life Event Ratings: An Independent Replication' in *The British Journal of Clinical Psychology* 20, 133–4. Leicester: The British Psychological Society.

Seligman, L. 1992. *Helplessness: On Depression, Development and Death* (second edition). USA: W.H. Freeman.

Szasz, T. 1991. 'Dialogue as Therapy'. Speech given at the Fourth Annual Conference of the Society for Existential Analysis. London.

Vacc, N. A., Wittmer, J. and DeVaney, S. 1988. *Experiencing and Counselling Multicultural and Diverse Populations*. Muncie: Accelerated Development Inc.

Winn, L. (ed.) 1990. *Power to the People*. London: King's Fund.

Index